My Yoga Road Trip

Navigating the twists and turns of life with yoga by my side

Clare Murray

Grosvenor House
Publishing Limited

The book cover is copyright to Clare Murray
Cover artwork and cover layout by
Stewart Shield and Jim Counsell

This book is published by
Grosvenor House Publishing Ltd
Link House
140 The Broadway, Tolworth, Surrey, KT6 7HT.
www.grosvenorhousepublishing.co.uk

A CIP record for this book
is available from the British Library

ISBN 978-1-83615-242-2

PREFACE

Embracing the practice of yoga. Join me on my unique journey as I continue to embrace my passion for yoga. When I took my first class on a borrowed mat, I had no idea that it would become the foundation of an adventure that would literally transform my life in ways I could never have contemplated. The teacher asked us to leave the world behind and be prepared to uncover an inner exploration, yoga being more than just a physical practice. In that moment, it became a sacred space where I could reconnect with myself, body, mind, and soul, finding a place of peace and calm. Then over a period of years, as my practice deepened, during retreats, courses, and travel I discovered the beauty of yoga philosophy, the many teachings of ancient sages, and many different styles of yoga.

So, to anyone facing their own trials and tribulations, I extend an invitation to embrace this gift of yoga, to share the practice in these pages to find a sanctuary of your own, a place of healing, peace, and resilience in this crazy world. Let this practice become your guiding light on the path to recovery and transformation, as we rise above life's challenges and become extraordinary. (A quote from my guru: "You're already great, now value yourself and what you do, project that, and let yourself become amazing.")

I'm grateful to all the teachers who brought me to this place and yoga into my life. From that first wonderful lady in her beautiful studio, and many teachers found at the gym who guided me through different styles of yoga, to the one-to-ones, the fabulous retreat teachers, not forgetting the many workshops and, of course, my guru. Thanks to these teachers, yoga has become my faithful companion and taught me that life's challenges – and there have been many – are not meant to break me but to shape me into a stronger, more compassionate, more awakened being.

Yoga has led me through the storms and shown me a better way to live. I truly do not know what would have become of me without yoga in my life.

MANTRA

My breath is my constant companion. When I feel anxious, I breathe deeply and I start to feel calm. My breath is my constant companion. When I feel anxious, I breathe deeply and I start to feel calm. My breath is my constant companion. When I feel anxious, I breathe deeply and I start to feel calm.

— unknown

I use this particular mantra often. It holds the power for me to stay centred and calm when at my most vulnerable.

BEGINNINGS

And so it begins. Approximately 30 years ago, amidst my whirlwind life, I found myself at a crossroads and a friend encouraged me to join her on a six-week Hatha yoga course. I must admit I knew nothing about yoga. At that time my days were filled with the responsibilities of being a mother, wife, daughter, sister, granddaughter, friend, managing a business, and running a home. These demands left little time for me, and the thought of committing to something different like yoga felt like a challenge.

At the studio, I felt both uncertainty and curiosity at the same time. I had always been physically active, mostly through the aerobic classes I'd attended with my lovely cousin. But the idea of stepping into the world of yoga seemed very much like venturing into unchartered territory.

As the first class began, I found myself surrounded by a diverse group of individuals, all seeking something unique from this ancient practice. The instructor, with her serene presence and an aura of tranquillity, radiated confidence. While she gently guided us through the postures and breath-work, I felt a subtle shift within me – a challenge to slow down and be still, and an ultimate sense of awareness. Yoga offered me the space for exploration where I could delve into the depths of my physical and emotional capabilities. And as those six weeks passed, I noticed amongst the chaos of my busy life that yoga became a place of sanctuary.

Stepping onto my mat, I could momentarily release the weight of responsibilities and find solace in the present moment. With each breath I felt the layers of tension and stress that had accumulated over the years slowly dissipate. I was able to find a space to relax; a place for self-care. The more I embraced yoga, the more I realised that it's not just a physical practice, but a philosophy that extends into life.

After the six weeks, I decided to continue my practice and started attending classes at the gym, ending up with different teachers at various stages of their practice of evolving styles.

Over the next few years, my yoga practice evolved as I explored different styles, from Hatha in the beginning, moving slowly from pose to pose, followed by Vinyasa Flow, and the strength of Power Yoga and my very first Jivamukti class.

I experienced physical flow, meditation, chanting, spiritual teachings, and I loved them all. My favourite classes were invigorating Vinyasa sequences, linking breath with movement, followed by more challenging sequences involving twists, binding, and balances. The music consisted of ancient Sanskrit chants and a mix of playlists, which added to the experience.

I decided to go on a yoga retreat – my very first – and immerse myself deeper into the practice of yoga and all that entails.

MY FIRST RETREAT

September 2004, I set off to Egypt. I'd always dreamt of going there to see the pyramids and Sphinx, and here I was with a fabulous group of yogis and yoginis on an amazing and exciting adventure.

We began with 108 salutations (flow of movements) to the rising sun on the sandy shores of the Red Sea. It was tough: 108 rounds of surya namaskar synchronising breath and movement, honouring the rising sun, followed by more challenging poses, achieving wheel, mastering firefly, and headstand for the first time.

One evening, finding stillness in meditation and holding a piece of coral picked up from the beach, we were asked to focus on the object and contemplate the words from the teacher, "What is your purpose?"

The question hung in the air; it seemed so simple, yet carried the power to change everything. I felt a flood of emotions rising within me, threatening to overwhelm my composure as I reflected on the roles I fulfilled in my daily life – work, wife, mother, daughter. Each role carried expectations and responsibilities, and a sob escaped my lips as I realised that I had lost sight of who I was and didn't know my true purpose. I had by choice become entangled in the web of societal expectations, losing touch with the essence of who I truly was. The weight of unhappiness and unfulfillment were buried deep inside me.

On the outside, I had a life that seemed so perfect, yet in that moment I felt empty. In the midst of my tears and some confusion, I realised that my purpose could not be defined by external roles or possessions, to fit into predefined moulds, or to fulfil societal expectations. I needed to find truth (satya), to be authentic. I realised that I had been seeking validation and happiness from external sources, but true contentment (santosha) could only be found within the true self.

I didn't have all the answers, and in that moment I was pretty shell shocked, but I knew my purpose would reveal itself with the knowledge that it's not about having everything or nothing, but about embracing the beauty of the present moment and being true to oneself.

With a newfound sense of acceptance, I wiped away my tears and took a deep breath. My journey ahead was uncertain but hopeful. I had the tools and the power to write my future story and discover the essence of who I am and who I could become. In that moment of vulnerability, I realised that it was okay not to have all the answers. My purpose did not have to be rushed; I would get there by embracing the journey of self-discovery.

We travelled along the River Nile – a voyage through time and the exploration of Egypt's ancient wonders, its temples and ruins telling their stories of past civilisations. Humbled when visiting the pyramids, I found myself in the depths of the great pyramid – a truly surreal experience. The air was somewhat stale and musty, and the walk through the low tunnel was stifling and suffocating. Some people turned back, unable to cope with the confined cramped space, but by staying calm and reciting my mantra, I did it.

What followed was amazing. Standing in the presence of the Sphinx and the pyramids – these symbols of strength and endurance – was a reminder that we too can withstand life's challenges and emerge triumphant.

The camels were everywhere. Naively, I allowed the camel keeper to manoeuvre me onto the back of one of the animals, and it took off with me. Thankfully, my friend shouted for the keeper to stop it, and my one and only camel ride came to an abrupt end, with the keeper shouting aggressively, asking for money I think, and our guide refusing to leave my side for the rest of the trip.

We then travelled into the bustling bazaars of Cairo and immersed ourselves in the vibrant, busy streets, mesmerised by the people and culture that surrounded us.

As the retreat came to a close, we bade farewell, carrying the lessons and insights that had transformed our lives. The inspired practice had awakened a desire in me to change my life, and it had given me the tools and courage I needed to move forward.

I returned home and subsequently separated from my husband.

"To move, to breathe, to fly, to float, to roam the roads of lands remote, To travel is to live."
— Hans Christian Andersen

UNRAVELLING

The chapter of my life that I'd nurtured and had held so much hope for now had come to an end. The unravelling of a marriage is painful for everyone – feelings of grief, confusion, and heartache all entwined. And I struggled at first to make sense of it all. Questions swirled around in my head: What went wrong? Could I have done something differently?

After seventeen years of marriage, emotions of sadness, anger, guilt, and a sense of loss fought for attention. Would I ever find solace amongst this turmoil?

Yet, amid the darkness, I discovered a flicker of hope – a different future and different choices. And as I began the process of ending my marriage, I realised that this chapter was just that – a chapter. And amidst my grief, I found the freedom to explore my interests and to discover what I like to do. With the support from friends, family, and, of course, yoga, I found opportunities to deepen my knowledge and truly discover who I am.

It became a time to deepen my knowledge for self-discovery and growth. As life is a tapestry of experiences, I now had the chance to reimagine mine, to redefine my path and pursue new possibilities, and boy did I go for it. At times it was difficult navigating my new role as a single parent, and I gained a new admiration for anyone struggling with the responsibility of solo parenting.

But yoga gave me the strength and the tools to face the challenges and changes ahead.

"There is nothing Permanent except Change."

— Heraclitus

SERVICE

As the school holidays approached, I was offered an opportunity for my daughter and I to assist my teacher with children's summer holiday yoga sessions. Eager to give back and share my joy of yoga with others, and with a sense of anticipation, we readied ourselves for the first session, preparing the room by setting up mats and props.

Working alongside the teacher, we witnessed the magic of yoga come alive in the eyes of these children, and their enthusiasm was infectious. The school hall filled with laughter as the youngsters embraced the stories, practices, and teachings of yoga, the lessons subtly planting seeds of mindfulness, empathy, and compassion within them.

When it was over, the teacher thanked us for our time and commitment, but we were the ones who felt enriched by the experience. Through serving others and witnessing the impact of yoga on these young minds, we had received the gift of purpose.

Now ready to embrace the suggestion of becoming a teacher myself, my teacher recommended the YogaBugs Training Course. I completed the application with a written reference, and on 15th May, 2005, I became a certified YogaBugs Instructor, completing the children's yoga teacher training course in London (my first ever journey to the capital alone, which in itself was a challenge).

Equipped with the tools and qualification to introduce yoga to young minds, to nurture their innate creativity and flexibility, I embarked on a new chapter in my life, teaching in schools and sharing the ancient practices of yoga with children.

I taught in several schools in the area, and the feedback from parents and teachers was positive, as they noticed improved focus and calmness in the youngsters. Encouraged by these successes, on 6th November, 2005, I expanded my qualifications further and completed the teacher training for older children, becoming a Yoga'd Up instructor.

The gift of teaching children is one which I cherish, and I am continually inspired by their willingness to embrace new experiences, approaching the practice of yoga with curiosity and playfulness.

This decision to become a yoga teacher set me on the path of purpose and fulfilment that I'd been looking for, allowing me to touch the lives of countless young souls and share the gift of yoga.

In each school, I witnessed the children's growth as they engaged with the practice. Their flexibility and physical abilities improved, but more importantly, they began to embrace the values of yoga – kindness, compassion and self-awareness. The photograph below is from a newspaper article, covering the introduction of yoga into local schools.

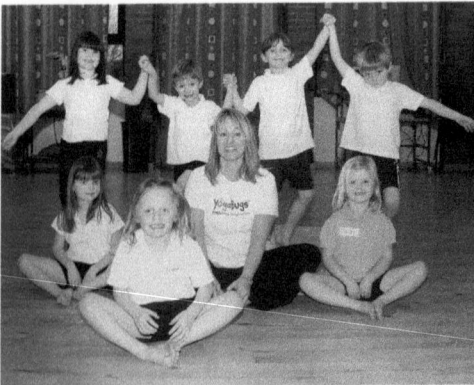

Teaching in a local school
Photo courtesy of ILIFFE Media Group Ltd

DEVELOPING A
DEEPER PRACTICE

Still working, but now teaching several times a week, I realised the importance of my own yoga practice. Eager to learn more, I continued to delve deeper and attended more workshops and retreats. They became moments of self-care as well as the expansion of my knowledge.

I enjoyed a weekend in a yoga centre in Cornwall (Tredardock), during which I experienced satsang (a gathering of like-minded individuals), and studied asana-poses, pranayama breath-work, meditation, karma lecture, silent walking-meditation, restorative yoga, obstacles to yoga-kleshas, physical alignment, and setting an intention for practice. Talks on the Yoga Sutras and Bhagavad Gita were all part of the weekend.

I met some fantastic people and felt a massive shift in my life – a realisation that through this practice, I could release the continuous stream of questions and worries that had been holding me back for so long.

My teacher gave me a card with the words of a mantra: *Lokah Samasta Sukhino Bhavantu.*

Translated, it means:

May all beings everywhere be happy and free, and may the thoughts and actions of our lives contribute to that happiness and freedom for all.

This is one of the most powerful mantras I have learned, and I repeat it often. I can't really describe in words just how much this mantra means to me, and how it helped on this particular occasion to get me through the events happening at the time. I can only describe its meaning and hope that you find what you need from the words, as I have.

MANTRA

Mantras are sacred words and phrases that vibrate when repeated over and over again. So, if you find yourself needing some mindfulness, positivity, and calmness, this mantra can become a useful tool.

Calmness: This mantra focuses on happiness and freedom for all, inspired by a sense of peace and tranquillity. When faced with challenges, recite this mantra and allow the vibration to find a place of inner calm and balance.

Compassion: The mantra's essence revolves around the well-being and happiness of all living things. Repeating it, you cultivate a compassionate heart and a sense of connection with others. In moments of conflict or frustration, the mantra reminds you to be empathic.

Mindfulness: Chanting and repeating this mantra brings you to the present moment, creating a space for self-reflection and peace.

Positive Intentions: This mantra carries the intentions of happiness and freedom; by chanting it, you align your thoughts with positive intentions.

I continue to embrace this mantra as one of my yoga tools. You may find, as I have, that it becomes a source of guidance and inspiration for you to continue on your journey of self-discovery and growth, and to live a life of purpose.

I often chant whilst riding my motorbike. It helps me to focus, be calm, stay present in the moment, and most importantly be safe.

TEACHING TEACHERS

The school teachers approached me with an eagerness to learn yoga themselves, and after my initial surprise, I made enquiries looking for an adult yoga teacher training programme that would fit in with my busy schedule. I chose a course with BSY (British School of Yoga) mainly because it was a correspondence course, with 200 hours of physical practice with your own teachers signing personal practice sheets, and two days of practical training plus written coursework.

I completed the diploma on 10th July, 2006, and the practical exam on 17th September, 2006 – two years after my return from the transformational retreat in Egypt. That set me off on another path: teaching yoga to the schoolteachers themselves, and then teaching yoga to adults.

On the Cornwall retreat, I met a lovely couple, and Simon embarked on teacher training around the same time in an Indian ashram, studying Sivananda. He taught for the Adult Education Authority and corporately in businesses in the area. When he asked me to cover some of his classes, I accepted with some trepidation, and the teaching of adults began in earnest.

As part of teaching adults, I was asked to complete a City and Guilds course in teaching, followed by my very first interview in years – with the Adult Education Authority. I actually got the job, one night a week, for which I had to produce a written teaching plan, objectives, outcomes, and reports, etc. I went on to teach at another local secondary school and gained even further experience, now teaching four adult classes a week alongside the children's classes.

During this time, I continued my own practice and attended retreats in Spain and France. I also continued with valuable one-to-one practices with the teacher who had encouraged me to become a teacher myself. She personalised these sessions to my individual needs, physical techniques, alignment with adjustments, and breath practices. I remain always grateful to this wonderful teacher who opened the doors to this amazing practice. She was there when I needed encouragement and picked me up when I was at my lowest. Thank you to my wonderful teacher for sharing your knowledge of yoga with me.

MALA

Mala – a Sanskrit word meaning garland – is used as a tool for meditation. I first encountered a Mala when Simon (friend and yoga teacher) came back from an ashram (spiritual place of retreat) in India with a string of Mala beads as a gift for me.

Years later, I now have a few Malas: one for chakra chanting and meditation; a Mala made up of rose quartz for travel (it's smaller); and two Malas that my dear student made with beads she brought back from India.

What is a Mala, and how do I use it? A Mala consists of 108 beads, and the purpose is to sit quietly and rotate each bead, counting one at a time whilst meditating. I use mine as a distraction from the constant chatter of my monkey mind. I hold the Mala in any hand and rotate the beads one at a time in-between my thumb and fingers, whilst inhaling and exhaling slowly.

Sometimes, I use the beads to keep track of how many times I've chanted a mantra or just simply to count. Remember, you don't have to be religious to use a Mala. I use mine as a tool to keep me focused during a meditation and to help with feelings of anxiety. My beads remind me of the need for peace and calm when facing the many challenges of life.

RETREATS

Om Mani Padme Hum – A Buddhist mantra – Jewel in the lotus of the heart. Repeated many times, this opens up the heart centre to love and compassion.

Aura Soma Yoga Retreat in the beautiful countryside of the Lincolnshire Wolds. It is a beautiful house in the heart of this county, offering lots of restorative yoga and relaxation, chakra yoga, kirtan (chants) Mantra, and an excellent Thai foot massage. What's not to like? Bliss.

The next retreat I attended was in Spain – at **Molino Del Rey, Andalucia.**

The retreat revolved around daily themes. The first day's theme was Ahimsa – non-violence and compassion towards all living beings, including oneself, cultivating kindness and understanding.

We studied karma yoga and acts of kindness towards others, acting with love and devotion, free from attachment to the fruits of our actions. Also, forgiveness for the burdens we carry, grudges, resentments, and unresolved emotions. As we released these heavy burdens, I experienced a new-found sense of lightness and liberation.

The principles of Dukha (suffering) and Sukha (joy) – the inevitable experiences of both as we learn to embrace the challenges and joys in life, the highs and lows, of the rollercoaster ride that is life, eventually finding the all-important balance.

Santosha – Contentment, reminding us to find peace and gratitude in the present moment, without constantly yearning for something else. The practice of Santosha leads us to an appreciation for the abundance already present in our lives.

The Kleshas – Affictions that cloud the mind. Through self-reflection and introspection, we identified patterns and gained the tools to move forward with clarity. Faith opens us to trust even in moments of uncertainty.

The exploration of Samskaras – Scars – allowed us to recognise and understand how the patterns of our past experiences have shaped us and how, with this knowledge, we can consciously reshape them allowing for growth new and beginnings.

This retreat was a real haven, a sanctuary with beautiful meditation caves that echoed with ancient wisdom. The centre also boasted the most enchanting Shala (studio) built into the mountain, creating amazing sounds and vibrations when chanting. Each day we gathered and immersed ourselves in the practice of yoga asana, breath-work and the themes of the day. Outside, the retreat centre pool became a place of rejuvenation, where we could cool off, while the meditation caves offered another escape from the heat of the day and a space to be silent.

An enchanting day was spent with fellow yoginis in majestic Ronda, the stunning vistas offering a glimpse into the heart of Spain's rich heritage.

This still remains one of my best ever retreat centres and was truly unforgettable.

FRANCE

A spooky old convent in the south of France. Sessions included Tibetan short-form yoga, Rishikesh series, Jivamukti yoga, Sivananda yoga, restorative sessions, yin sessions, pranayama, breathing practices, Ujjayi (sometimes known as the ocean breath), Bhramari (bee breath), talks on the Bhagavad Gita, yoga Sutras, Kirtan (chants), mantras.

Though the practice of Karuna, compassion, through heart-opening lessons, we embraced our vulnerabilities and extended compassion to every aspect of our being. The theme of humility reminded us to remain grounded and open. Some of us did an evening talk or guided a meditation, and I shared a poem chosen from a book my mother gave me, *The Creed of My Heart*. Poetry for the Spirit, titled "Adversity" – by Michael Dillion – the poem speaks of resilience, transformation, and the strength that lies within us all. As I read, I felt a deep connection to the words.

This retreat brought us all together with an emphasis on sharing our practice, our unique stories, walks, meals, kirtan (songs, chants), evenings spent sharing our reflections, experiences, and insights. Each person's unique perspective offered fresh insights and diverse approaches to embracing the teachings from the Bhagavad Gita and the Yoga Sutras and applying them to our lives beyond the retreat.

Sharing the poem with the group brought about a degree of vulnerability in me. I was nervous, but the shared experience was important to me, and with support and encouragement we discovered that despite our diverse backgrounds and the differences in our lives, there was a common thread that united us all: the yearning for knowledge beyond our own, the safe environment without judgement or competition. This was a space created for us to be our authentic selves, free from pretence and expectations, and it's with gratitude that I've had the opportunities to attend – and still do – these wonderful retreats with the most amazing shared stories connecting us through yoga.

I recommend taking notes, as you never know when you may refer back to dates, experiences, and perhaps your thoughts at that time.

I've always been a note taker, and every year – usually on my birthday – my mum buys me a little notebook (paper blanks). They come from an independent local book shop and fit into any bag. So, I always have one with me. It's these little journals, plus various clippings of all my notes pertaining to yoga workshops I have attended, which have given me the opportunity to share my experiences with you.

This is a shared recipe from one of my journals:

Sante Biscuits: 4oz butter, 2oz sugar, 6oz flour, 1tsp baking powder, 3 heaped tsp condensed milk, 3 drops vanilla essence.

Cream butter then add all other ingredients. Grease a tray, roll mixture into small balls and flatten.

Bake 20mins max at 170 (can add 2oz dark chocolate or nuts). And enjoy.

"The reward of a thing well done is to have done it."
— Ralph Waldo Emerson

ACCIDENTS

There have been quite a few, but I'll keep to the ones that relate to this period in time.

In picturesque Chamonix, France, after a scary but stunning journey up the mountain in cable cars, followed by a chairlift, skis dangling, yoga breathing engaged, beautiful untouched virgin snow, fresh crisp air, beautiful blue skies, and the most majestic views of mountains I'd ever seen. I traversed carefully down the first slope, then waved my fellow skiers past as we all approached the mogul slope, happy to slowly traverse at my own pace. Unfortunately, fate had a different plan for me that day, as a reckless skier crashed into me, leaving me slumped in a heap of snow. Unable to ski and in a lot of pain, I limped down to the connecting slope. And at the medical centre the swollen knee revealed a suspected ruptured ACL (Anterior Cruciate Ligament).

During an MRI on my return home, evidence of an old fracture in the distal end of my femur from a previous accident (yes, there have been a few) emerged. With that came the future potential for arthritis if left untreated. I was told that surgery was the only way forward, followed by six weeks of non-weight-bearing recovery.

The accident left me feeling extremely vulnerable, as I lived with my teenage daughter in a small village, so we would need some help. Fortunately my children stepped forward with unwavering support and care. My son and his then girlfriend moved back home and became a pillar of strength, as did my wonderful sisters-in-law, brothers, cousin, parents, and lovely friends.

During my recovery, I found myself revisiting a passage from a yoga book, involving an ancient story that mirrors the unpredictable nature of life. I'm relaying it from memory.

It's the tale of the farmer who caught a wild stallion. His neighbour exclaimed, "You're so lucky to have caught that beautiful stallion." The farmer responded, "Maybe, maybe not." When the farmer's son broke his leg trying to tame it, the neighbour commented, "That's so unlucky." Once again the farmer responded, "Maybe, maybe not." Soon after, war broke out and the army came to enlist the young men of the village. They bypassed the farmer's son with the broken leg, and the neighbour remarked, "You're so lucky." "Maybe, maybe not," came the reply from the farmer. That night, there was a great storm, and all of the animals escaped. The neighbour predictably says, "You're so unlucky." And as expected the farmer replies, "Maybe, maybe not." The horse then comes back with a big herd, and the neighbour says, "You're so lucky." And so the tale continues.

The story of the farmer has stuck with me over the years, reminding me of the impermanence and uncertainty of life. Accidents and challenges in life are inevitable, but the essence of yoga teaches us to embrace each moment. We may not always understand the unfolding events, but within each experience lies the potential for growth and wisdom.

Yoga became my anchor during this time of recovery, and with my new degree of patience and perseverance I navigated the journey back to strength and mobility. I was discharged immediately from physiotherapy and told to just continue with my yoga.

The accident had not only tested my physical strength but also taught me lessons in surrender, resilience, and the art of letting go. There was so much I couldn't do; just making a cup of tea was a challenge. I feel lucky to have amazing people in my life who stepped in and helped just when I needed them.

I continued to work from home, with work dropped off to me, and I started some online courses. Yoga therapy was one of them, due to my interest in yoga as a holistic method for healing, both physically and mentally, delving deeper into the therapeutic benefits of various yoga techniques, asanas, pranayama, meditation, relaxation, and their potential for healing.

The journey into basic counselling was a natural extension of my desire to support others. And the course deepened my understanding of active listening, empathetic communication, and holding the space for individuals to explore their emotions and experiences.

I found myself drawn to the idea of integrating yoga therapy and counselling into my teaching. The knowledge and insights gained during this time became invaluable in my own healing journey as well. Looking back at all my painful experiences, I see that what may have appeared as unlucky at first, became a chance for growth, expansion, learning, and exploring new passions. It was a reminder that life's twists and turns often lead us to opportunities.

By the way, I wouldn't wish injury or any form of hardship on anyone as a way to seek personal development. There are many paths to self-discovery and growth that don't involve adversity of this kind. So go forward, experience workshops, retreats, courses, and seek guidance from mentors, teachers, and books. May our journeys be guided by curiosity, compassion, exploration, and most importantly passion. And may we continue to seek ways to deepen our knowledge and understanding of the world around us and our connection to it.

Funnily enough, as I hobbled around on crutches showing people around my house while still very much recovering, my house sold and the challenge began to find a new home, and another new beginning.

"The secret of change is to focus all of your energy, not on fighting the old but on building the new."

— Socrates

THE FIVE TIBETAN RITES

Five rites – said to be practised by Tibetan Monks – are thought to hold the secrets to a healthy long life by regulating the endocrine system, using the circulating energy of the body. This story was told by an English Colonel who travelled to Tibet. Many years ago, I was given the book *The Eye of Revelation* – written by Peter Kelder in 1939 – which shows the five Rites of Rejuvenation.

They seemed so simple when I first practised them on a retreat, and I didn't really think about the possible benefits at the time. However, I now feel they have become an empowering sequence that play an important part of my routine.

Start slowly, with fewer repetitions to begin, and always take medical advice before practising any new routines.

1st Rite

Stand up straight and stretch arms to shoulder height, palms facing down. Spin to your right, keeping your eyes open; spin for 21 repetitions on the same spot. To begin, maybe start with 5 and build up to 21. Children love this one. (Oh, and don't forget to breathe.)

2nd Rite

Lying on your back, place your hands alongside the body. On an inhale, lift the legs and head at the same time. Exhale and lower. Repeat 21 times. To begin, maybe start with 5 and build up to 21. And perhaps bend your knees if you have any back issues.

3rd Rite

Kneeling upright, with hands placed on the back of the thighs, inhale and drop the head back, opening the chest. Bring the head and chin back on the exhale. Repeat 21 times – again, start with 5 and build up to 21. Do not practise if you have neck issues; instead, seek medical advice. I personally never complete 21 of these, happy to do just 5.

4th Rite

Sit on the floor, legs out straight. Inhale, pushing palms into the floor. Bending knees, slide feet towards hips and inhale lifting the bottom off the floor into a table top position, keeping fingers pointing towards the feet, exhale and slowly come back to seated. Repeat 21 times, or start with 5 and build up to 21. Avoid if you have wrist problems; instead, seek medical advice. I prefer to do 10.

5th Rite

Start in upward facing dog with toes curled under, Inhale to downward facing dog, then exhale to upward facing dog. Repeat 21 times, or start with 1 round and slowly build up to 21. I find 10 plenty at the moment.

Adapt the repetitions to what feels right for you. The benefits:

Improves circulation, coordination, strength, and fitness.

Improves sleep, anxiety, and energy.

PURIST: No, it's not for me.

The beauty of yoga for me lies in its inclusivity and acceptance of all individuals, regardless of lifestyle choices or beliefs. Yoga for me is not about conforming to a rigid set of rules or being a "purist"; it's about embracing authenticity, being true to ourselves, and finding balance and harmony in our lives. We all have our path, our individual journeys, which aren't about perfection but perhaps embracing imperfections, moving towards self-improvement and growth instead.

Being a yogi, yogini doesn't mean giving up all the things you enjoy or conforming (my least favourite word) to what someone else thinks you should or ought to be. To me it means living life with mindful awareness. Yoga teaches balance in all aspects of life: enjoying a glass of wine with a delicious meal of choice; joyfully experiencing favourite activities and hobbies without judgement. Yoga encourages us to let go of judgement and comparison, to release the need to fit into any specific mould, honouring our true selves and remembering you are perfect just as you are. You can embrace uniqueness and honour choices authentically.

After I got divorced, I accepted an invitation to a charity clay pigeon shoot. I really enjoyed doing something which was totally alien to me, having never tried shooting with a shotgun before. After a fantastic afternoon enjoying the challenge of the competition, I decided to apply for my own shotgun licence.

I'll never forget the chap who came to interview me and check that my gun cabinet conformed to the required specifications. He asked me about my personal relationships and appeared very interested in my divorce. But I must have said something right, because I got my licence and off I went gun shopping, then to the local shooting ground to learn how to shoot safely.

Since then, I've enjoyed many wonderful afternoons shooting clays, and when I met my present partner we shared many great times in the beautiful outdoors, at various shooting grounds. I was fortunate to receive some excellent tuition from my partner's best friend, who happened to shoot for England. I never really improved much, but that wasn't the point. What's important is to try things, to explore, to experience things that take you out of that place of comfort, and find your full potential.

Eager to embrace new experiences and adventures, I took on another challenge. My business involved selling motorcycles, and having taken my Compulsory Basic Training (CBT) many years before, I decided it was time to pursue a full motorcycle licence.

One day, a lady walked into the showroom enquiring about a Suzuki GSXR 750 motorcycle and asked to deal with me. After some negotiation, we agreed a price for her part exchange, and I made an impulsive decision to purchase her Honda NC30 400 motorcycle myself. The lady was so small in stature, her toes barely touching the ground, but she was huge in courage and personality, leaving me totally in awe of her. With her in mind, I decided to take the next step, and what followed was a week-long intensive motorcycle course – first to pass my theory test, then renew my CBT – shortly followed by the full test. This included the tricky U-turn, which I struggled to do without putting my feet down (an instant fail).

Along came the day of the test, and the challenge of the U-turn was upon me. Thankfully, I did the U turn without putting my feet down, but halfway through the test, whilst weaving through traffic, I left my instructor behind. I returned to the test centre expecting that I had failed. But surprise, surprise, I passed. I was so chuffed that I gave him a big hug – needless to say, he was horrified.

The point I'm making is we should grab opportunities as soon as we can. And it's in those moments of doubt and insecurity that my yoga breath and the power of self-belief shines through.

"Perfection. Better to live your own destiny imperfectly than to live an imitation of somebody else life with perfection."

— Bhagavad Gita

What is perfection? What does perfection look like to you?

Maybe accept the concept that you are perfect just as you are right now and celebrate the beautiful tapestry of life. Fill it with experiences, adventures, and share your love of life, no matter what that entails.

Being a "yoga purist" is not what matters to me. What matters is sharing my love of yoga and hopefully inspiring you to embrace your own yoga journey with uniqueness, honesty, authenticity, and most importantly acceptance and compassion.

So, if you want to raise a glass of wine, enjoy the flavours of life and continue to share the magic which is yoga with me, authentically and unapologetically, and remaining – of course – "imperfectly perfect".

"Let the beauty that you love be what you do!"

— Rumi

This is one of my classes taught around this time:

Set an intention for your practice, embodying flow, and creating conditions in which prana (life-force) can flow freely throughout the practice.

Start lying on your back, with feet on the floor at the outer edges of the mat, bent knees touching, arms beside the body, palms up, fingers relaxed (constructive rest).

Breath practice (pranayama), extending the exhalation breathing only through the nose, for 3 minutes.

Inhale and take one ankle/heel of foot to the outside of the opposite knee. Apply a little pressure, pushing the knee/leg to the floor, and hold for a breath. Repeat on the opposite side (pinwheel).

Inhale one knee into body, exhale and squeeze; inhale and repeat with the other knee, exhale and squeeze; inhale both knees together, exhale and squeeze, holding onto shins (apanasana).

Exhale knees over to the floor, easy twist, with knees moving each side and shoulders remaining on the floor. (Support the knees with a block if needed.)

Slow bridge 5 repetitions (setu bandasana). Push feet into the floor. Inhaling, lift hips and arms towards the ceiling; exhale the arms to the floor behind the head; inhale arms back to ceiling; and exhale hips and arms down.

Inhale, and rock up to seated cross legs, if possible. Place one hand onto the side of the head and apply pressure, whilst exhaling to gently stretch the neck, then inhale the head back to centre. Repeat each side.

Inhale to lift arms, and exhale to forward fold. Inhale back and change cross of legs and repeat neck stretch, and forward fold.

Child's pose (balasana) – pushing buttocks back to heels, bring forehead towards the floor, taking a few deep breaths. (Modify by separating the knees, or placing a block in-between thighs and calves.)

Kneeling salutation sequence – 5 repetitions, from kneeling to extended child's, to inhale onto all fours lifting tail bone and face to cow, then curl toes lift knees to exhale down dog, inhale dropping hips towards the floor up dog, exhale to down dog, then inhale back to cow, exhale pushing buttocks to heels extended child's, and inhale back to kneeling. (See drawings of sequence later in the book.)

Down dog, hold for 5 deep breaths. (From hands and knees, lifting knees off the floor, straighten legs, and push into the heels.)

Sun salutation B – 2 repetitions. From mountain standing, inhale and lift arms, bending the knees; exhale to a forward fold; inhale, lift the chest slightly, fingers to the floor, shins, or block; exhale, jump or step back to four-limbed staff (plank to floor), lower to the floor exhaling. Then inhale, lift chest, pushing into hands cobra; exhale to down dog; inhale, step right foot forward in-between hands; turning left foot in slightly, lift arms into Warrior 1 (front knee bent, arms either side of ears); exhale and step back, repeating the sequence on the other side.

Standing balance sequence – inhale and lift knee to hip height, taking opposite hand to outside of raised knee; exhale to twist in opposite direction. Repeat other side.

Vinyasa flow to the floor, (Inhale lifting arms, exhale forward fold, inhale lift chest to half forward fold, exhale jump or step both legs back to plank, and lower to the floor) resting forehead on backs of hands, and take a few breaths.

Locust pose (shalabhasana) – Take your arms down beside the legs, with the palms facing the floor, extending the toes, stretching the front of the ankles. Inhale, lifting one leg; exhale down. Repeat with the other leg. Then inhale lifting both legs; exhale down. Repeat, now inhaling lifting both legs, both arms and head; exhale down and repeat (continue with single legs and arms as a beginner).

Seated heroes sequence – kneel, then sit back into the space in-between feet (or onto bricks/blocks), alternatively single leg with one leg extended forward. Hold for a few breaths.

Seated forward fold (legs in front aligned) to table top. Push into feet and lift bottom off the floor, do 4 repetitions. Inhale to lift, exhale to lower.

Reclined twist (easy twist), inhale bringing knees into the body, exhale knees to one side, hold and breathe for five deep breaths then repeat on the other side.

Relaxation.

Place something warm over your body and find a comfortable position (savasana or constructive rest) and close your eyes. Have a fidget and perhaps take off your glasses or anything which may make you feel uncomfortable.

Take your awareness to the breath, and just notice how the breath is moving your body. Continue to allow your body to sink, relaxing more and more with each exhalation. Become aware of the feet, and inhale moving the toes, then exhale finding stillness in the feet and ankles; bring awareness to the calves and knees, and inhale tense then exhale and relax calves and knees. Bring awareness to the thighs; inhale tense, then exhale relax the thighs; become aware of the buttocks, inhale tense, and then exhale releasing the buttocks. Become aware of the lower back, inhale and draw the navel towards the spine, pushing the small of the back towards the floor, then exhale and release the lower back.

Bring awareness back to the breath. Take a big inhale and notice the ribcage expand back into the floor, then exhale and release, allowing the shoulders to sink and relax into the floor. Bring awareness to the hands resting on the floor, inhale and make a fist, exhale and release, relax the hands and arms. Inhale, bringing awareness to the neck and throat, exhale and swallow, releasing the neck; move the tongue around the mouth. Inhale and squeeze eyes tightly closed, then exhale and allow the eyes to be gently closed; inhale and draw the eyebrows together, then exhale and release the forehead; inhale and become aware of the back of the head, and exhale the weight of the head on the floor.

Now, just notice the breath. Has it slowed down? Is it smooth and regular? Just follow the breath, the inhale, the exhale, and continue to follow the breath as you allow your body to relax fully.

Rest in this position for a few minutes.

Now begin to move the feet, then stretch arms and legs, hug both knees and rock over onto the right side of the body, push to a comfortable seated position, hands in prayer. Notice how you feel. Take your time to open your eyes.

Namaste.

"Remember that not getting what you want is sometimes a wonderful stroke of luck."

— Dalai Lama

I was extremely fortunate to have some wonderful yoga teachers, and one in particular invited me to a local art/photography exhibition. Jeremy Hunter is an award-winning photographer, and I was particularly drawn to his work – the Tibetan Monks meditating in the snow. In fact, I was so inspired that I bought it and arranged to meet the photographer, who signed it for me. It hangs as a reminder of a time many years ago and the inspiration that came from a photograph.

In Labrang, East Tibet, the Monks use the ancient art of Tum-mo meditation – an advanced and deep meditative state to raise body temperature using both the breath and visualisation. It's a demonstration of the power of the breath and visualisation, and a reminder that we too can harness these tools to provide improved health and well-being in our own lives.

I think this is the Prayer of Saint Francis of Assisi. I first heard it as a song, but I prefer the translation of the original:

"Lord, make me an instrument of your peace. Where there is hatred, let me bring love. Where there is offence, let me bring pardon. Where there is discord, let me bring truth. Where there is doubt, let me bring faith. Where there is despair, let me bring hope. Where there is darkness, let me bring your light. Where there is sadness, let me bring joy..."

It continues with another verse. Check it out on the internet, or try the Serenity prayer. I like to begin my meditation with a prayer or mantra, it helps to set both my mood and intentions.

ACCIDENT

2nd October, 2008

On my way from covering a yoga class at the gym for a friend, I found myself involved in another accident. This one was a turning point in my life; one that reminded me of the preciousness of each moment and the importance of living with gratitude, authenticity, and a poignant reminder that life is filled with unexpected events.

The accident left me trapped and unconscious in the moment of impact. Blurry upon awakening, I had a surreal experience first of peace and detachment, a feeling of surrendering to the unknown, and a sense of calm and acceptance. But with a jolt, reality struck me as I became aware of my surroundings and the terrifying sensation of being trapped.

Panic surged through me. I couldn't find the door handle, nothing was in the right place, it was dark, and the eerie sounds were unsettling, whirring and hissing, the ominous smell of smoke lingering in the air. Terror took over as I struggled to make sense of my surroundings, still totally disorientated. I tried to move but was trapped by my seatbelt (which thankfully saved my life), and in the darkness I couldn't find a way to release it.

Take a breath and calm down, I told myself. I managed to calm my breath and first moved my toes, felt my legs and arms, then moved my head. Relief flooded through me, and I finally managed to release the seatbelt and fell into the roof of the car, realising for the first time that I was upside down. Strangely, I felt no pain just panic. The thought of being trapped in a burning car filled me with terror, and in the chaos of that moment I knew

I had to act fast. As I called out for help, a voice in the darkness responded, then a man appeared struggling with the door but only managing to open it slightly. I got my arm out and said, "Just pull me."

He finally managed to free me from the wreckage, and I took a deep breath and tried to scramble my way up the slope but collapsed. Relief and pain took over. I remember shaking, unable to move, only managing to breathe. Blood was visible on my hand and a sharp pain pulsed in my hip.

The car had not caught fire but was unrecognisable. The experience left me reminded of the fragility of existence, and the unpredictability of the path we walk.

The accident was another turning point in my life – a reminder to cherish every breath, and now knowing I'm not afraid of death. In that moment, I had felt so peaceful. And it's in those moments of fear and vulnerability that we find a wealth of strength within us. Through adversity, we find resilience.

In the aftermath of this accident, recovery became my primary focus – a journey that tested not only my physical strength but also my emotional resilience. The physical wounds healed, but the emotional scars lingered, leaving me feeling vulnerable and fearful of the future. During these moments, I turned to my yoga practice, which reminded me to trust and embrace change with an open heart, to accept the impermanence of life, and to find strength in surrendering to the flow of existence. Through asana, I found my physical strength; through pranayama and mantra, I found a way to calm my emotions and panic.

As I write this chapter, I am reminded of the resilience that lies within us all, the capacity to adapt to heal, and to move forward with forgiveness. The accident is a reminder of life's fragility but also a gift, a catalyst for growth, an opportunity to move forward and head down a different path. May my experience be a reminder to embrace change with an open heart, to find strength in vulnerability, and to trust in the magic of transformation that lies within us all.

As I stood at the crossroads of my life again, I felt a surge of courage and determination within me. The accidents had been harrowing, but they had also served as a catalyst for transformation. It was time for a new beginning, a fresh chapter that revolved solely around my passion for yoga.

With a heart full of conviction, I made the decision to take a leap of faith and let go of my other role and move away from the business I'd been a part of for so long – a shift from a world of engines and finances to one of asanas and mindfulness. It was a moment of liberation and trepidation.

As I embraced the uncertainty that lay ahead, I knew it wouldn't be easy, but I found solace in the teachings of yoga. After all, it had guided me so far to trust the practice that had been my refuge so many times. I had to let go of the identities I had held onto for so long and now embrace just being a yoga teacher.

In those early days, I faced doubts and insecurities. Was I making the right choice? Would I be able to sustain myself financially? But amongst the uncertainty, there was a new sense of purpose. As I embarked on this new path, I found support and encouragement from those who believed in me – my partner and family, dear friends, and the yoga community. Their unwavering belief in my potential gave me the courage to keep moving forward, even in moments of doubt.

The journey was not without challenges, but I approached each one with the resilience I had cultivated through my practice.

I sought guidance from my teachers, and I continued to deepen my knowledge through workshops and retreats. Teaching yoga became more than just a profession; it became a constant exploration of myself, each class an opportunity to share the gift of yoga.

May my journey be an inspiration for those who are at their own crossroads and encourage you to take that big step forward with courage and faith.

I chose to include the following picture, as a visual reminder of the devastation caused by the action of one person – though not intentional. It was an accident; the driver of the car that hit me simply fell asleep.

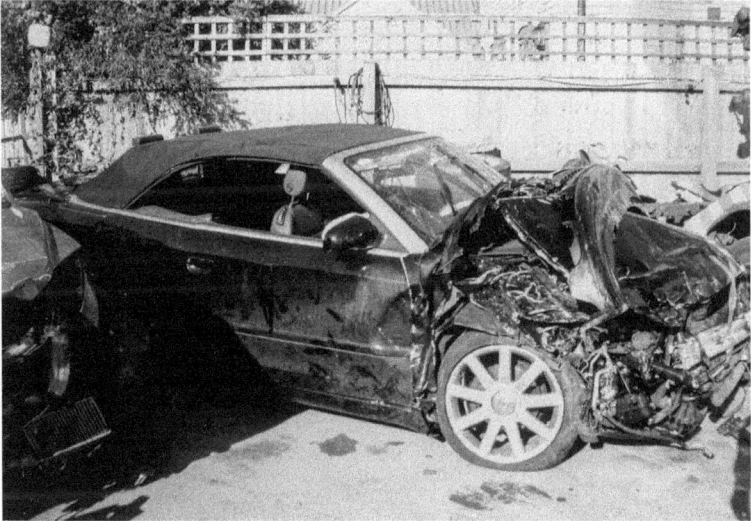

VAIRAGYA – NON-ATTACHMENT

Meaning: When one does not grasp onto things, the reason for one's life, why one is born, and what is to become of them, becomes clear.

Patanjali

Patanjali's teachings remind us that the practice of non-attachment is not about giving up all material possessions, desires, attachments, and all that gives you joy. But to overcome the distractions and desires of the material world to encourage us to attain a clearer vision of our true nature and purpose.

The story of the greedy buzzard

After consuming a large meal, the buzzard grabbed the remains in its claws and flew high up over the trees, where it was spotted by some hungry blackbirds. They gave chase, bombarding the buzzard and grabbing at the remaining food. Even though the buzzard was struggling to hold onto the remaining food, its full belly making it hard to fly, it stubbornly refused to let go. But the blackbirds were persistent and continued their attack until the buzzard could no longer hold on. Finally it let go and the remaining food fell to the ground with the blackbirds in pursuit, leaving the buzzard alone in the sky.

The buzzard found it's freedom from suffering by letting go of greed.

(Source unknown, found in my notes)

We have two pairs of buzzards living in the nearby copse and I often watch them flying over our house with blackbirds in hot pursuit.

Doesn't a good clear-out make you feel great? Bringing better organisation from decluttering saves time, allowing you to find what you want more quickly. And letting go of old, unused stuff creates space. It can be a way of letting go of the past, therefore allowing us to embrace the future full of new adventures and new experiences with fresh energy.

We are encouraged throughout life to work hard and save hard for our future, and there's nothing wrong with that, but again it's about choices and perceptions. After a heated discussion with my partner, he made a comment, "Really, Clare, how much more do you need?" The comment made me reflect on the words of Patanjali, the recent accident, my travels... What more do I need? Thinking of the greedy buzzard. What could I let go of? And off I went to meditate on that.

"We need much less than we think we need."

— Maya Angelou

NAVIGATING TRAUMA IN THE HOSPITAL WARD

As I lay in the hospital ward, the open wound in my hip a visual reminder of the accident the day before (2nd October, 2008), my head throbbed with a pain so intense that I could only imagine it like the ferocity of a migraine. The agony vibrated through every inch of my body, each pulsating throb intensifying my discomfort even more.

A drip hung from my arm – a lifeline tethering me to medication and the bed. Battered and bruised, I lay unable to move. Vulnerability wrapped itself around me like a shroud. Across from me lay a young woman, burdened by pancreatitis and a daunting battle with alcohol, her eyes sending a plea for me to listen, to share the burden. And in the quiet corners of the ward, her story unfolded the worries of a mother with two small children and the challenges she faced.

Beside her, in the other bed, an elderly lady was tethered to a machine that echoed its constant rhythmic beep – a reminder of the fragility of life. The lady next to me, hidden behind closed curtains, grappled with the indignity of a leaking stoma bag. The smell hung heavy in the air, a contrast to the sterile environment of the hospital.

The elderly lady's monitor alarm went off, a cry cutting through the ambient sounds of the ward. The noise quickly became a form of torture, amplifying the helplessness that permeated the ward. I rang the bell for assistance, concerned for the lady who clearly couldn't help herself. The response, however, was far from helpful. A nurse arrived, her demeanour sharp and aggressive, a contrast to the vulnerability surrounding us.

"What is it?" she demanded, with gritted teeth.

I explained in a quiet voice that the elderly lady's alarm had been sounding persistently, and she looked unconscious.

The nurse's response, cold and dismissive, was, "I'll get to it when I'm ready," brushing off any urgency with callous indifference.

In that moment, anger and frustration threatened to boil over, and despite my own incapacitation and through clenched teeth but loud enough for her to hear, I replied with an insult. Yes, I lost my cool and temper, my anger overwhelming me, and my head began pounding even more aggressively. I never saw that nurse again.

This is a snapshot of my experience – on this occasion with this particular nurse – of the unspoken battles within the hospital ward, the silent screams of pain and frustration that often go unheard. It's a narrative of vulnerability in the face of an indifferent system, a reminder that within the sterile walls of health care, empathy and compassion are as vital as the medicines administered.

Later that day, after a shift change, a lovely nurse went above and beyond duty, giving me a bed bath. She handled everything with such gentleness, making sure we were all comfortable. Finally, the poor lady's stoma bag got sorted out, and the nurse even found time to bring some magazines for the young lady opposite. It just goes to show that there are nurses out there who truly have a calling for this work, having empathy and understanding. I was so grateful for her that day.

So, thank you to all the great nurses out there. And to those not so great, don't add to someone's trauma, and remember to treat people how you would want to be treated yourself.

"I am not what happened to me, I am what I choose to become."

—Carl Jung

TIME TO STUDY

After being asked for advice on diet, I thought it wise to further expand my knowledge on the subject. So I completed the CIBTAC diploma in diet and nutrition on 19th August, 2009, followed by a Yoga Therapy online course on 8th September, 2010.

Recipe for soup: Leek and Potato.

Ingredients: 1 onion, chopped; 225g-8oz potatoes, cut into cubes; 3 leeks, chopped; 55g-2oz butter; 850ml-1 1/2 pints vegetable stock; salt and pepper; garlic (optional); creme fraiche or double cream (optional).

Melt the butter in a large saucepan, then add the chopped vegetables and cook for a few minutes or until soft. Add the stock and bring to the boil, then reduce to simmer for 10-15 minutes. (Optional, add garlic). Liquidise the soup and season, add creme fraiche or double cream if required. Serve with some homemade crusty bread.

I started going annually to Mind, Body, Soul Weekends, and explored lots of different styles of yoga and interesting seminars on health.

These gave me my first taste of Kundalini yoga, Fire yoga, Power Chi yoga, Vibrational healing, many healing talks, a mantra workshop, and meditation sessions. These were affordable weekends which offered a wide variety of classes and subjects to choose from.

I have many fond memories of sharing these weekends with both past and present friends.

MANTRA MEDITATION – SO HUM

So – I am   Hum – That

Find a comfortable position to meditate, resting hands either in the lap or perhaps in a mudra of your choice.

Take a few nice deep breaths. Repeat the mantra silently to yourself to begin.

Inhale So... Exhale Hum... Repeat with a chant: Inhale So... Exhale Hum... Repeat for 5-10 minutes.

Increase the duration of the meditation as you become more comfortable. You can use different words as a mantra – e.g., a simple In and Out, or Inhale Calm, Exhale Relaxation.

Benefits: calming and relaxing for the mind and body.

HYPNOTHERAPY 2010-2011

Whilst delving into yoga therapy, the course briefly touched on the subject of hypnotherapy. The idea of combining it with yoga seemed like a natural extension of my yoga practice. After some research, I found a year-long accredited hypnotherapy course and arranged a meeting with the tutor. She was warm, knowledgeable, and passionate about the power of the mind and its potential for healing through hypnosis.

The tutor shared her experiences of how hypnosis brought about changes in people's lives, releasing emotional traumas and overcoming fears. Throughout our conversation, I could sense the genuine care and dedication she had for helping others. It was evident that this was the next step. I'd found my teacher with her background in nursing and I knew I'd be in safe hands. With that in mind, I enrolled and committed to the course.

Becoming a qualified hypnotherapist, armed with the knowledge and techniques I had acquired through the course, I stepped into the role, ready to support others. As I began my practice as a hypnotherapist, I found myself humbled by the vulnerability and courage of my clients. Through the power of hypnosis, I witnessed the transformative potential of the human mind, as clients opened up their subconscious, uncovering the roots of their challenges, and navigating through traumas, limiting beliefs, and emotional blockages to become empowered to make positive changes.

Each session, I witnessed massive shifts in my clients' lives. And I felt a sense of gratitude for the trust my clients placed in me and a profound responsibility to guide them through the sessions with no judgement or expectation. I found the union of yoga and hypnotherapy enriching, giving me the confidence to take the next step and continue with more in-depth yoga training.

CREATING A SAFE ROOM

Every client creates their own safe room, and this is a good place to start any session.

Remember, before any session of Hypnotherapy, you are always in control and can stop and open your eyes whenever you choose.

Begin by finding a comfortable and quiet place to relax, where you won't be disturbed. Once you are settled, close your eyes. Remember, you are safe and always in control. Take five slow deep breaths in and out; now just watch the breath, and focus on the rise and fall of your chest. Eyes still closed, feel the movement of the breath in your body and relax more deeply, allowing your body to continue to sink and relax. Now think of a safe word – the first one that comes to mind – and imagine a door in front of you. It has your name on it. There's a lock, and only you have the key to open it. You open the door and walk in.

Now create your SAFE room:

Is there a carpet in your safe room? If so, what colour is it? What does it feel like under your bare feet? Is the floor is tiled or wooden ? Become aware of the texture. What colour are the walls? Are there any pictures or paintings hanging on the walls?

There's a bed in front of you, with blankets and cushions. What does it look like? Create a comfortable, cosy bed and find yourself lying on it. Sink into the mattress and relax, always in control. What colour are the cushions? What fabric is the blanket?

Notice how comfortable you feel – warm, cosy, and completely safe.

NOW, repeat your safe word, and know that any time you need to go to your safe room, you just close your eyes, relax, repeat your safe word, and go to your safe room and relax.

Bring yourself back to the present moment, feeling relaxed and calm. Take five slow deep breaths, slowly allowing your eyes to open until you are wide awake.

May my journey as a hypnotherapist inspire others to embrace the healing potential within themselves and to walk the path of self-discovery.

Affirmation

> *"Every day, in every way, I am getting better and better and better."*

Emile Coue, French psychologist and pharmacist, was a pioneer in positive thoughts and healing using autosuggestion.

YOGA ALLIANCE TEACHER TRAINING WITH STEVE

5th Jan 2013, 220hrs

First question asked: What does yoga mean to you?

The yoga alliance teacher training with Steve in Sheffield was a journey filled with great anticipation and a touch of apprehension as it marked the first long journey I had undertaken on my own since the last accident. Again, I leant on my pranayama practice, chanted mantra, and with nerves fluttering in my tummy, I arrived to be greeted by a wonderful atmosphere amongst the other participants.

With energy fizzing in the room, the training was set to be a deep dive into philosophy, chakras, asana practice, and teaching the methodologies of yoga.

The first question posed by Steve resonated deeply within me: "What does yoga mean to you?" In that moment, my mind drifted back to the accidents, the moments of vulnerability, and the journeys back to recovery, and there it was. My answer came effortlessly, as if whispered: Yoga to me meant recovery and purpose. Yoga had been my refuge during my darkest times; it had cradled me in its embrace, offering a sanctuary. The practice provided the tools to navigate through my physical and emotional challenges.

Among the many practices yoga has gifted me, Nadi Shodhana (alternate nostril breathing) stands out as my go-to breath. This simple pranayama has the power to calm my panic every time. As the days throughout the year of training unfolded, I immersed myself in the teachings, eagerly absorbing the wisdom generously

46

shared by Steve and my fellow participants, each practice, each discussion, taking us deeper into the practice.

Steve, a true yogi — a guru, even (I don't use that word lightly) — embodied the essence of yoga in every fibre of his being. His compassion and non-judgemental nature created a safe and nurturing space for us to explore and grow, and boy did we. He walked, talked, lived, and breathed the true wisdom of yoga, and his presence was a source of inspiration for us all.

I can still hear his soft, accented voice singing the Gayatri Mantra with the gentle strumming of the guitar in the background. And I still have the CD recording Steve made for us. The power of sound — the crystal bowls he played as a treat for us, added a touch of magic. Vibrations resonated through our bodies, calming our minds and inviting us to sink deeper into relaxation and stillness.

Finding Steve was an amazing stroke of luck, a serendipitous encounter that added depth to my yoga teaching, his sessions taking us beyond the physical postures to dive into the heart of yoga philosophy and spirituality.

As I reflect on the yoga alliance teacher training, I am reminded of the beautiful tapestry of souls that came together in that space, with each participant bringing their unique story and experiences that can never be replicated. It was an honour to be a part of this group. Steve treated each one of us with care and respect, guiding us with patience and grace. His ability to hold space for our struggles and triumphs made me feel understood and supported.

As the training came to an end, the lessons, the memories, and the wisdom shared will remain with me forever. The privilege of spending time with Steve was a gift that would continue to inspire us in our personal practices and our continued journey as yoga teachers, the impact of his teaching extending into every aspect of our lives.

May the light of Steve's teachings continue to shine bright in our hearts, and the memory of his gentle guidance and support inspire me to continue walking the path of yoga with compassion and dedication, with love and gratitude. I dedicate this chapter to Steve: your impact on my journey of yoga and recovery will forever be treasured. I honour your influence in every class that I teach. Thank you.

In memory of my guru.

"Live each moment completely, and the future will take care of itself."
— Paramhansa Yogananda

Nadi Shodhana: Alternate nostril breathing practice

Start in a comfortable seated position (blow your nose) and take a few deep breaths. Close your eyes.

Take your right hand in front of the face, and close the right nostril with your thumb. Inhale deeply through the left nostril then pause, closing the left nostril with the ring finger. Release the thumb, then exhale through the right nostril and pause. Then inhale through the right nostril, pause, and close the right nostril with your thumb. Open the left nostril and exhale, then pause.

This completes the first round of Nadi Shodhana.

You can do as many rounds as you want, but I would start with five rounds and build up to ten. Notice how you feel and tailor your practice accordingly.

If you can't breathe fully through your nose, just close your eyes and visualise yourself breathing alternately through the nostrils as instructed above.

STORY OF THE MONK

Two monks walking along a riverbank come across a woman sitting by the shallows, not daring to cross. The older monk asks if she wants help to cross. "Yes, please." So he lifts her onto his back, carries her across the river, puts her down, bids her farewell, and continues on his journey.

The younger monk mumbles under his breath and, after walking for some time, can no longer contain himself. He asks the older monk, "Why did you carry that woman across the river?"

The older monk replies, "Why are you still carrying her?"

How many thoughts do we carry with us every day?

How do we expect to focus on the moment when our minds are so full of stuff?

Could we let go of any of that stuff?

"To the quiet mind all things are possible."

Meister Eckhart

'Yogash Chitta Vritti Nirodha'

This comes from Patanjali's yoga sutras, translated as 'Yoga is the cessation of the fluctuations of the mind'.

The essence of this sutra is to convey that the practice of yoga aims to quieten the fluctuations of the mind (quieten the monkey mind) and bring it to a state of stillness and tranquillity. When the mind is free from the constant stream of thoughts, desires, and distractions, we can experience a deeper sense of peace, clarity, and self-awareness. If we can integrate this into our lives, we can navigate the challenges we face with greater clarity and resilience.

This brings me to an example of this in my life:

It was on one of my motorcycle adventures — a road trip across Spain with my partner. When riding on the motorway outside Seville in the scorching heat and heavy traffic, suddenly my partner encountered a problem and lost the full use of his gears, with no choice but to stop at the side of the motorway against the Armco barrier. The situation was dangerous, with cars and lorries speeding by, and in those nerve-wracking moments we jumped the barrier to some safety.

I needed to quieten my racing heart and jumbled thoughts, and to focus on what truly mattered in that moment. I took a deep calming breath, closed my eyes, and — holding my rose quartz Mala tightly in my shaking hand — I started to chant the words silently, "Yogash chitta vritti nirodha." I did this over and over again for a few minutes, until I found the clarity and a sense of peace amongst the chaos of my surroundings.

When I opened my eyes, feeling much calmer and with my breath and heartbeat now slowed, I noticed a slip road approximately 200 metres away. And further down was a Repsol garage (petrol station). Suddenly the path became clear and a solution emerged. We could limp in first gear along the hard shoulder to the garage, safely assess the damage, and find some shade whilst having a cold drink. By the way, my partner's go-to solutions are more practical — cable ties and gaffer tape seem to solve all his problems.

It happened again on an adventure to Italy, via France and Switzerland, across the Alps and down to the most beautiful

Italian lake. It was our first time taking the motorbikes through the Channel Tunnel. My partner on his new motorbike, me on my trusty steed, the trip offered exciting roads, beautiful scenery, and challenging mountain passes. After a fantastic, but arduous, three weeks of travelling, it was time to return home.

On the M11 back in England, my partner's bike suddenly lost all power. He slowly veered dangerously across the three lanes towards the hard shoulder, rolling to a standstill, explaining through the intercom what was happening. What followed required much patience, as we waited for the recovery vehicle.

I made the decision to return home alone, trying to dismiss what could have been a fatal outcome. My partner's sudden move across a busy motorway had been terrifying, and maintaining my composure had been a challenge. But I focused on staying calm and breathing steadily, using my internal mantra to see me safely home again.

Now, I'm not suggesting that everyone needs to break down on a motorway or dangerously veer across three busy lanes to practise mantra and breath-work, but this is just an example of the many situations I've found myself in where yoga has come to the rescue.

The teachings of yoga have become my constant companion, guiding me through life's ups and downs, helping me stay calm and focused, giving me the strength to face any challenges that come my way. As I continue this journey as a motorcycle-riding yoga teacher, I'm grateful for the interconnectedness of my passions and how each enriches the other. I've learned that yoga for me is not about fitting into a particular mould of what I should be; it's about embracing all aspects of who I actually am and finding balance, joy, and serenity in all that I do and all that I continue to enjoy.

May my experiences inspire others to embrace their passions, whatever they are, to live with authenticity, joy, and a whole lot of adventure.

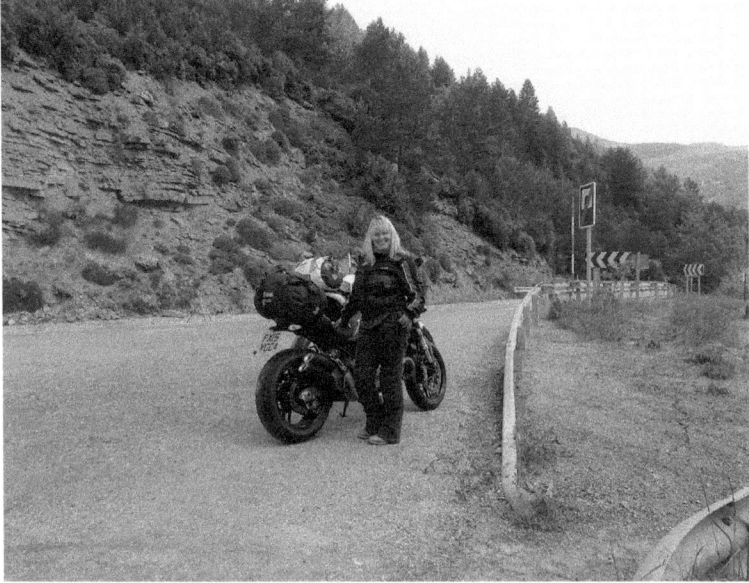

Spain on motorbike

Like water in the stillness of a lake, which mirrors the sky and trees only so long as its surface remains undisturbed, the mind can only reflect your true image when it is tranquil and wholly relaxed.

I wrote this in a journal many years ago and can't remember where I first heard it. But I share it regularly, as it reminds me of the importance of a calm mind.

REFLECTIONS FROM THE HYDROTHERAPY POOL

One of my first jobs after college was in the hospital's physiotherapy department, where I helped in the hydrotherapy pool and with the stroke and amputee patients. It was here that I encountered many patients facing extraordinary challenges.

Three patients in particular stand out in my memory. The first was a fourteen-year-old girl grappling with a form of rheumatoid arthritis, which had already tested her young spirit. My role was actually really simple yet meaningful — to care for her after her hydrotherapy sessions. I would wrap her in warm blankets and provide her with a comforting hot drink and a chat. Her gratitude was immense, and her words echoed with the profound difference our treatments made in her life. Her resilience, smile, and grace in the face of adversity were a source of inspiration to me.

The second patient was a man who had endured an unimaginable gunshot wound to the back that forever altered the course of his life. Yet he embodied remarkable strength and an unwavering spirit that allowed him to carry on with life's challenges without complaint or self-pity. His determination to persevere was a lesson in resilience that left an enduring impression on me.

Lastly, there was the elderly gentleman — a man whose manners and grace were simply impeccable. His interactions were a testament to the enduring power of kindness and courtesy. Even amongst his own trials, he extended warmth and respect to those around him, leaving a lasting lesson in good manners and respect.

At the tender age of eighteen, my year in the physiotherapy department provided me with a profound insight into the struggles that some people must confront on a daily basis. It served as a reminder that, by comparison, I had been granted a significant head start in life.

The experiences of that year instilled in me a great sense of gratitude, which has remained with me throughout my personal traumas, reminding me of the enduring strength of the human spirit and the transformative power of empathy and compassion. These were profound lessons learned in the presence of those who face adversity with grace and resilience.

From what I witnessed, the healthcare professionals, including nurses, caregivers, and physiotherapists, provided invaluable support, care, and compassion to individuals facing illness, injury, and the challenges they face every day. Their dedication and selflessness not only make a difference in the lives of patients but also inspire gratitude and admiration in those who witness their remarkable work.

MIND, BODY, SOUL WEEKEND

One of my lovely students (Sue) organised a group of people from the gym to go on these weekend events. As I mentioned earlier in the book, I went on a few of them and really enjoyed being a participant.

This particular weekend started with a fabulous teacher utilising the chakras and pranayama to influence and increase the flow of vital energy. We went through the chakras, using asana and pranayama for each one — a really lovely class — followed by a session of Budokon flow and flexibility. Budokon is a dynamic blend of traditional yoga asana and martial arts, building on the traditional hatha yoga practices in a non-conventional, challenging way.

I enjoyed the opportunity to explore a very different approach. Yoga Nidra and the Art of Meditation was a theory and practical session giving great tools to combat stress and train the mind. These weekends included sessions of: Yoga, Tai Chi, Zumba, Yin Yang, Shiatsu, Qigong, Chiball, Pilates, Acupressure, and Emotional Freedom Technique. There were also talks on subjects such as: sugar, the effects on the body; Release Me; angels; the Chinese 5 Elements; seasonal well-being; face yoga, and many more.

It was an opportunity to try different classes and listen to subjects we may have never come across. And of course, we could chill out with like-minded people over breakfast and evening meals. Most of the weekends offered treatments and spa facilities, so all round it was great fun and I have lots of fond memories.

Transformation

"If you desire a glorious future, transform the present."

Pantanjali

Think about how a chrysalis changes into a beautiful butterfly, and know that you have the power to transform yourself. A butterfly signifies transformation — a reminder that we can all embrace change.

These weekends were an opportunity for gym members to explore many different styles and to give them the confidence to try something new.

RETREAT IN NORFOLK

18th October, 2014

Leading my very first retreat day in Norfolk, the tranquil studio over-looking the serene lake was a joy.

As the participants arrived, we had tea and a brief chat, detailing the timetable of the day. The morning session started with a vibrant invigorating ninety-minute vinyasa flow. The studio space was filled with the sound of breath and movement as we flowed from one pose to another, syncing our movements with the breath.

After the morning practice, Tanya prepared a fabulous lunch — a nourishing and delicious spread of homemade veggie dishes.

Next, we put on our walking boots and set off on a guided walk amongst the beauty of the lakes and woods that surrounded the studio, followed by a ride around the lake in a speedboat.

The afternoon session was slower, more yin style, with restorative poses followed by a long relaxation. The slow, mindful practice allowed us to release tension and find stillness. After a day of yoga, we indulged in the luxury of a hot tub session.

That first yoga retreat day in Norfolk had been a resounding success, and for me — the facilitator — it was a rewarding experience witnessing the participants embrace the practice and connect with each other, finding moments of serenity amongst their busy lives.

Timetable of My Retreat

The day starts at 10am with arrival teas, juices, introductions, and a short talk.

11am – Yoga Vinyasa flow style in the studio overlooking the lake.

12.30 – Lunch, all home-made fresh local vegetarian food.

1.45pm – Guided walk, or free time to relax in the beautiful garden by the lake; optional boat ride.

3.30-5pm – Yoga Yin style with restorative/supported poses and meditation, followed by relaxation.

Optional speedboat ride - use of bikes - hot tub.

Example of what I teach on a Retreat Day/Weekend

The warm-up sequence, followed by a Yin Practice:

Start in a comfortable seated position, cross legs if possible. Take awareness down towards the earth Muladhara Chakra - Mula - Root, Adhara - Support, Root into the Earth, every sitting pose activates Muladhara. This chakra anchors us to the earth, providing stability and strength. Visualise the colour RED. Think about strength, and engage Mula Bandha (root lock). Hold onto the knees and exhale allowing the back to slump, dropping the chin into the chest, then inhale straighten the back, bringing the chin back, move with the breath for five rounds.

Move awareness to the pelvis and just focus on this area. Svadhisthana Chakra – that which is one's own abode, gateway of the Moon. Think of the words joy and creativity, and visualise the colour ORANGE, or think of holding a juicy orange in your hand. Smell the orange and feel the texture of its skin. Now place your hands on the knees and circle the hips, bringing awareness to Svadhisthana.

Bring your awareness higher towards your navel. Manipura Chakra - city of jewels, gateway of the sun. Think of a flame providing light and heat, digestion and fire. Imagine the colour YELLOW warming the skin, and come into a seated twist, bringing hands to one thigh and turning the head to look over the shoulder. Bring your awareness into the chest cavity. Anahata Chakra — The un-struck sound; gateway of the winds. Think of the words compassion, empathy, and love, and imagine all the different shades of GREEN in nature and allow them to spread across the chest and into the heart. Extend your arms out in front of the chest, then inhale open them wide, exhale close the arms, dropping the chin, then inhale open again, lifting the chin, and repeat 5 times.

Move awareness to the throat — Chakra Vishuddha — to purify; gateway of time and space, communication, speech. Think about the colour BLUE — a pale blue sky — and let this colour spread into your throat. Healing opens up your ability to communicate. Neck rolls, dropping chin to chest, back straight, exhale roll the chin to the left, inhale roll the chin back to centre, then exhale roll the chin to the right, and repeat.

Move your focus to the forehead, in between eyebrows — Ajna Chakra, Third Eye — to perceive, gateway of liberation, intuition, clarity of thought. Think of a SAPPHIRE and imagine placing it onto your brow in-between the eyebrows to open up your intuition. Eye exercises: squeeze the eyes shut, then open wide, look right then left, right then left, right then left, squeeze the eyes shut, open wide, look up then down, repeat (only move the eyes, not the head), close the eyes and rub the hands together until the hands become warm, then cup them over the eyes and absorb the heat/energy.

Moving awareness now to the crown of the head — Sahasrara Chakra, Thousand Petalled Lotus Gateway of the void. Imagine a halo of bright WHITE light, and exhale forward fold. Hold for five breaths and repeat changing the cross of legs. Close your eyes and notice how balanced you now feel.

Take a deep breath in through the nose and out through the mouth, Haaaaaaaaa. Repeat 3 times.

Tanyas Coconut and Date energy balls were so good that I found a recipe online and played around with it:

Ingredients: 20 pitted dates; 1 cup of desiccated shredded coconut (unsweetened); 1/4 cup of raw cacao powder, or cocoa powder; 2 tablespoons of water.

Set aside some of the coconut. Add dates, coconut, cacao powder, and water to a food processor. Mix thoroughly, then take a large spoonful of the mixture, roll into a ball, and roll in the coconut until covered. Place onto a baking tray and repeat the process until all of the mixture has been used.

Place the balls into the freezer for a couple of hours, as this allows them to become firm. You can either remove and store in the fridge or put them into a container and keep in the freezer.

Enjoy.

APAN MUDRA

The Mudra I regularly use is APAN MUDRA (Energy Mudra)

This Mudra is said to help remove toxins from the body, assisting with urinary issues. It is associated with the element of wood and connected to the liver, bringing purification and balance to the body.

Find a comfortable position and take both hands, palms facing upward. Bring the thumb and two middle fingers to touch, then extend both little and index fingers. Hold for 5-10 minutes, or longer if you can. Repeat every day.

A nice easy **Mantra Meditation** I first encountered on a Retreat many years ago:

Sa Ta Na Ma — touching each finger one at a time, reciting Sa Ta Na Ma, starting for 3 minutes and progressing to 12 minutes or longer.

Sa - Infinity

Ta - Life

Na - Death

Ma - Rebirth

Letting go of the past and becoming your true self.

You can find mantras and chants on YouTube or Spotify.

INDIA, MY FIRST VISIT

9th Jan, 2015

My first trip to India was a thrilling adventure from the moment I stepped onto the plane at Heathrow. First stop was Mumbai, then the Jivana Plantation, Goa. The long journey was made more enjoyable by my trusty iPod loaded with meditations and chants that kept me calm and relaxed during the flights.

Upon arrival in Mumbai, I was blown away by the vibrant energy, sounds, and smells. I couldn't wait to dive into the array of classes and workshops at the yoga centre. The days were filled with a diverse range of yoga styles and practices.

The first body art sequence flowed gracefully through various asanas, a hot yoga-styled class followed by walks to the beach, morning flows followed by partner flow, and then an interesting power workshop with a shaman, which gave us profound insights. Soul-cleansing hypnosis took me on an inner journey, unlocking hidden potentials and clearing away mental blocks, Sivananda-style yoga infused me with a sense of peace and harmony, while the London-style hot yoga class challenged and invigorated my practice. Evening Yin yoga provided a restorative end to the day, allowing me to sink deep into relaxation, followed by a brilliant night's sleep. Inner peace workshop facilitated introspection, and a visit to the magnificent Banyan tree left me in awe of its majestic presence and profound symbolism.

We departed the plantation early one morning, heading by train for an eight-hour journey across country to Hampi. The station was crowded and chaotic and I found myself separated from my group in a carriage with the locals. Although initially daunting, it turned into an incredible opportunity to immerse myself in the rich culture of India.

The people were incredibly friendly and eager to share their stories and culture with me. One person spoke English and acted as a translator, bridging the communication gap. I was offered food and entrusted with holding their baby.

The train journey lasted eight hours, and I relished every moment, soaking in the sights and beautiful scenery, listening to all that unfolded around me. It is awe-inspiring how quickly we can adjust to new surroundings and situations, from bustling, unfamiliar cities, the tranquillity of nature, or embarking on a life-changing journey. Our ability to adapt and embrace the unknown is truly remarkable.

Ancient and mystical Hampi is a land filled with enchanting temples and a unique blend of tradition and adventure. After our exhilarating train journey, our exploration led us to cross the river in a fascinating traditional round boat. As we ventured deeper into Hampi, we encountered delightful surprises at every turn, witnessing an elephant being washed in the river, cows randomly wandering along the roads, and monkeys everywhere. We shared some exciting rides in the rickshaws, which we nicknamed the wacky races (an old cartoon).

Throughout our journey, we met children, their bright eyes filled with curiosity and wonder as they stared at my blonde hair. Interacting with them was a heartwarming experience, and they taught us valuable lessons about joy and the power of connection beyond language and cultural differences.

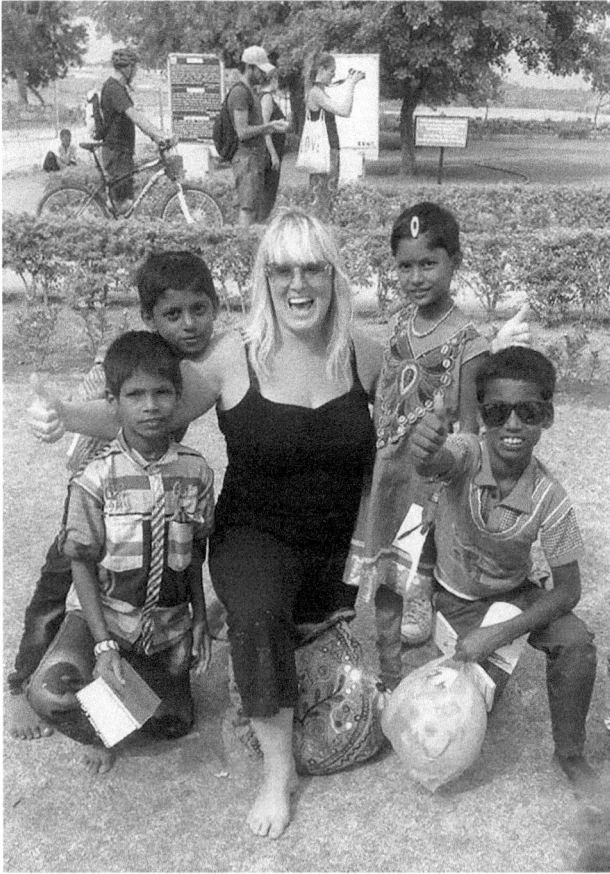

Our guide Hanuman, just turning seventeen, told us his prize possession – apart from his cow, of course – was his little old motorbike. He wanted to see pictures of my bike and children and was in awe of me and my life, while I was in awe of him and his beautiful smile. When I told him he had the most beautiful smile and was always smiling, he replied, "Why would I not be smiling?" Why indeed. A simple life in a beautiful place surrounded by lovely people.

One evening, Hanuman guided us on a spiritual journey up the six hundred steps to the Hanuman Temple. As the sun began its descent, the monks filled the air with the chanting of prayers, creating the most amazing atmosphere of serenity and devotion. Mischievous monkeys surrounded us, making the experience feel surreal. It was definitely the most spiritually moving experience of my life.

Hampi was a place of contrasts: paddy fields, temples, exhausting yet invigorating, chaotic yet serene, poor yet rich, ancient yet evolving. There were unforgettable moments of stillness and reflection, some filled with laughter, others with awe, all enriched by the graciousness of the locals.

The last day in Hampi started with a nature walk through the sprawling Hampi Boulders, covering 52 acres (no, we didn't walk it all). Our path led to caves across a bamboo bridge, channelling our inner Indiana Jones and feeling like explorers. Climbing to the top of the cave, we were rewarded with breathtaking panoramic views and it was as if time had stood still. We continued to the Elephant Temple, where we were graced with the presence of the painted elephant – a magnificent creature adorned with jewels and painted with colour, who bestowed a blessing upon us.

The journey through Hampi had been truly transformational, a pilgrimage full of memories which we would carry in our hearts. Thank you, Hampi, for the gifts you bestowed upon us.

As we began our journey back to Mumbai at 5.30am, little did we know India had another surprise for us. The flight was cancelled, but "That's just India" became the chant. Taking yogic breaths, we remained calm, and after many hours of delays and detours, I found myself back in Mumbai in a luxurious 5-star hotel.

The contrast between the opulence of the hotel and the experiences I'd had in Hampi and the slums in Mumbai left me feeling a mixture of gratitude and guilt. We were invited on a slum tour where we got a glimpse of what life is like for those who live there. Yet, despite the challenges they face every day, they appeared remarkably happy and content, their smiles radiating warmth and appreciation for the little they have.

During the tour, we were graciously invited into one of their homes – a small, basic dwelling which was extremely cramped but clean and tidy. A lady dressed in the most vibrant colours approached me and our guide translated her words of gratitude for our visit. I was so moved by her appreciation, and I thanked her for allowing us into their homes and sharing their hospitality. Later we took a train across Mumbai to the iconic Gateway of India.

Back at the hotel, I couldn't shake the impact of the slum tour and the sharp contrasts of wealth and poverty in Mumbai. The areas surrounding the hotel were no-go zones, a reminder of the stark disparities that exist.

As my time in India came to a close, I reflected on the many experiences that had enriched and expanded my perspective. India had gifted me with moments of awe, adventure, and self-discovery, but it also highlighted to me the realities of inequality and social challenges. The most profound aspect of the people living in the slums was their lack of complaint or moaning, and their pride. It made me reflect on how often we take our own privileges for granted and focus instead on what we lack rather than appreciating the abundance of what we have. In the face of adversity, they smile and find contentment in the moment.

Their attitude served as a humbling reminder to be grateful for the blessings in my life and to find contentment in the present moment. It showed me that happiness doesn't always come from material possessions or external circumstances, but from cultivating a positive mindset and embracing life with an open heart.

The people in India taught me that true wealth lies in the richness of our relationships, the depth of our connections, and the joy we find in the little things. Their ability to find happiness despite their challenges inspired me to be more mindful of my own outlook on life and to approach each day with a sense of gratitude and appreciation.

As the plane took off, I looked out of the window and bade farewell to the enchanting land that had taught me so much. Back home, I embraced the familiar comforts with the desire to return one day with my partner. India had left an indelible mark on my soul, forever shaping the decisions yet to come.

"Always laugh when you can; it's cheap medicine."
—Lord Byron

ANOTHER MIND, BODY, SOUL BREAK...

This time, we joined stress management and goal-setting workshops, and participated in a more detailed Face Yoga session.

Along with Budokon and Capoeira yoga dance — very dynamic and challenging, igniting a sense of strength, agility, and fluidity — there was a great diversity of styles, always offering something unique, sparking our curiosity. Encouraged by these workshops and retreats, I decided upon another course and enrolled in a Restorative Yoga training course.

RESTORATIVE TRAINING

8th May, 2016

The restorative course at Camyoga, Cambridge, was a fantastic four days in which I deepened my understanding and practice of restorative yoga.

The course provided me with a comprehensive foundation in this healing and rejuvenating practice. We began by diving into anatomy and physiology, exploring how restorative yoga affects the neuroendocrine system and the subtle energy within our bodies. Understanding the scientific basis behind restorative yoga allowed me to appreciate its therapeutic benefits on a physiological level. As various asanas were explored, I learned how to modify and adapt postures to cater to individual needs and limitations. The focus on alignment and props emphasised the importance of creating a safe and supportive, comfortable environment during restorative practice.

Throughout the course, I had the opportunity to analyse and experience sample restorative yoga practices. And as we stepped into the teaching assessment, I was encouraged to cultivate my unique teaching style and voice while staying true to the essence of restorative yoga.

The course provided invaluable experience and insights. Throughout the four days, I engaged in fruitful discussions, shared insights, and learned from each of the participant's experiences. The sense of community and support among the group created a nurturing and enriching learning environment, enhanced by the two fabulous teachers with their incredible wealth of knowledge.

I like to include a restorative pose at the end of each class I teach.

My favourite go-to is supported fish (matsyasana), with a bolster when possible or bricks if not.

Relaxing the breath, opening the chest, it's great for releasing tension in the shoulders — which I think we're all in need of — followed by Constructive Rest for Relaxation.

Come to a seated position and place the bolster or bricks in alignment with the spine. Lay back on the support, allowing the hands to rest on the floor (palms up), with the shoulders releasing towards the floor. Hold for 3-5 minutes. Roll onto the right side of the body and remove the bolster or bricks. Come onto the back, bringing knees together and feet wide apart (constructive rest). Relax for 5-10 minutes.

TURNING 50

Turning fifty and embarking on a safari in Tanzania was a dream come true — a celebration of life, and a testament to the adventurous spirit that yoga had nurtured within me. As I journeyed over Kilimanjaro, and through Lake Manyara National Park, the Serengeti, and the Ngorongoro Crater, I was truly in awe of the magnificent wildlife that surrounded us.

Armed with my new camera, I captured breathtaking images of lions, elephants, giraffes, and an amazing photo of a cheetah yawning — all in their natural habitat. The game drives were filled with excitement and wonder, reminding me of the beauty and diversity of our planet. The hot air balloon ride over the Serengeti, with a magnificent sunrise of the most amazing colours, was a magical experience that also tested my fear of heights.

As the balloon lifted us high into the sky, I felt a mix of trepidation and exhilaration. I briefly closed my eyes and, holding my Mala tightly in my hand, I took some slow, deep breaths and silently repeated the mantra, "I am safe, I am safe", finding the strength to overcome my fear and embrace the experience fully. I'd practised some self-hypnosis, working on my fear of heights, and it enabled me to fully embrace the breathtaking views below.

We followed the trails left by hyenas, cheetahs, lions, and elephants, and it was so magical — my childhood dream of seeing these wonderful animals in their natural habitats, doing what nature intended. The experience included a champagne breakfast in the bush, which was a wonderful start to a perfect day and a fabulous way to celebrate turning 50. Seeing the big five all thriving in their natural environment, camping in the bush that evening, listening to the wonderful and truly unforgettable sounds of the lions, elephants, and wildebeest, was truly unforgettable.

However, the adventures weren't over yet. We continued on our journey, and another challenge awaited me on the beautiful island of Zanzibar, where I agreed to try scuba diving. Breathing underwater was a concept that had always intimidated me, but I was determined to face another fear. With the guidance of a skilled instructor, I submerged and, following instructions, we passed the first part of training in the pool and progressed to the ocean. Now seated on the edge of the boat, ready to fall backwards into the sea, I submerged.

My heart was racing, but focusing on my breathing just as yoga taught me — calm and slow, calm and slow, calm and slow — gradually the fear subsided to be replaced by a sense of wonder and amazement at the vibrant marine life surrounding us. Scuba diving offered a unique perspective of the underwater world.

Through these experiences, I realised that the tools I had cultivated in my yoga practice — mindful breathing, grounding mantras, and embracing challenges with an open heart — were not limited to the mat. They could accompany me on every adventure, enabling me to find peace and courage in even the most unfamiliar and seemingly daunting situations.

As I stood on the cusp of my fiftieth year, I felt an overwhelming sense of gratitude for the transformative power of yoga. It has not only filled me with physical and mental strength but also gifted me the resilience and courage to embrace life's uncertainties and explore the world with an open mind. Through all these moments, the essence of yoga guides me, inspiring me to seek adventure, embrace challenges, and cherish every precious moment of this beautiful life.

"You are never too old to set another goal or to dream a new dream."

—C. S. Lewis

NEGATIVITY

I had a situation that really got to me. I may be a yoga teacher, hypnotherapist, psychotherapist, and I consider myself a well-balanced and confident person, but this situation really got under my skin. A person from the gym kept making negative comments about the way I looked several times a week, every week, for months.

I didn't really take much notice to begin with, but after hearing negative comments about my appearance over and over again, it actually started to make me feel negative. It was like their words had this power to influence how I saw myself, and I found myself avoiding this person, not because I didn't like them but because their negative comments started to affect me.

It is strange, but not uncommon, how people sometimes feel the need to share their comments about the way you look. Maybe the first time they said it, they genuinely thought they were being helpful! But when repeated week after week, it makes you wonder. What was the point? Was it meant to be rude or even abusive? I mean, are people that oblivious to how they are making others feel? You can choose, as I did, not to engage with that kind of negativity and delete their words as unimportant.

There's a Buddhist quote that really resonates in this situation. From memory it goes something like: before you speak, ask yourself three questions — Is it true? Is it kind? Is it beneficial?

It's like a checklist before saying anything. Perhaps just thinking about whether what you're about to say passes these criteria can really make you re-evaluate what you're about to share, what impact your words may have on that person, and if it's helpful.

This experience has made me realise that negative comments about appearance can really mess with your mind. It also taught me the importance of setting boundaries and communicating how you feel. If this happened now, I would challenge what someone was saying and ask them to please stop commenting on how I look. If someone's comments — whatever they are — consistently bring you down, step back and surround yourself with people who lift you up, and maintain a positive and healthy environment for yourself.

Looking back on that situation, I realise that those negative comments about me were more about the person saying them and just their opinion, perhaps projecting their own stuff onto me. We can't be responsible for everyone's insecurities or issues, and some people just can't be helped no matter how much you try. People's behaviour often reflects their own inner struggles, and it's unlikely to be about you.

It taught me the importance of not taking things too personally and being compassionate, even when others are being negative or unkind. It's also a reminder to be patient, because we don't always know the whole story. In saying that, though we still need balance and while persistent negative comments can bring us down, constant praise or flattery can also have its pitfalls. Too much praise and compliments can inflate our ego and make us overly self-centred.

That brings me to the concept of Ahimsa — non-harming, excessive praise or ego can harm our sense of humility and authenticity. While it is wonderful to receive positive feedback and appreciation, it's important to balance this with a healthy dose of constructive criticism. Respect yourself.

"Stay away from negative people, they have a problem for every solution."

—Albert Einstein

As a yoga teacher, I've encountered a few negative comments, and another that stands out was, "I don't like Clare's yoga because she isn't spiritual." That's okay, not everyone resonates with my style of yoga. But what struck me was the label of "not spiritual". What does that mean?

It made me reflect on what spirituality means to me, and I realised that my spirituality isn't defined by beliefs or rituals. It's about connecting with myself and others, experiencing compassion and empathy, doing yoga, helping people by listening, writing a journal, repeating affirmations, and meditation. I believe that true spirituality is an intrinsic part of life, whether we're consciously aware of it or not.

In response to this comment, I pondered the notion of not being liked, or that perhaps this person didn't connect with my teaching style, and both of those reasons are perfectly fine. However, instead of simply accepting that fact, they felt compelled to vocalise themselves with a comment that felt more like an insult.

Patanjali sutra — when disturbed by negative thoughts, we should cultivate their opposite.

By cultivating attitudes of friendliness towards happiness, compassion towards suffering, delight toward righteousness, and calmness toward wickedness, thoughts become cleansed and the obstacles to self-knowledge are lessened.

So, rather than dwelling on the negativity, I choose to focus on the positive connections I've forged through yoga. Ultimately, my path is to share the gifts of yoga with authenticity and compassion, and I know that it will resonate with those who are open to it. As for the rest, well, I respect their journey and choices. After all, yoga is about finding our own paths and honouring our individual perspectives.

A positive mind remains optimistic about life.

A negative mind remains just negative about everything.

Lion pose — Simhasana:

Channel your energy and release tension. Find your inner strength by letting go of negativity.

Start kneeling, with hands on your thighs. Inhale deeply, then exhale, bringing hands forward to the floor, look up, stick out the tongue, and roar like a lion.

Inhale, sit back onto the heels, and repeat 2-5 times.

I usually start with a little roar (lion cub), followed by a female roar, then a full-on, all-out roar. This posture strengthens the neck, throat, and voice. It also helps to reduce any pent-up emotions, reducing stress and anger.

If you struggle to kneel, try placing a small cushion under your knees. Sometimes I teach lion as a seated breath practice, or when I feel the energy in the room is low. This pose never fails to make me smile. It's hard to be miserable when smiling.

Give it a go and see how it makes you feel.

PEA AND STRAWBERRY HEIST

My childhood was a fantastic time. I was a happy, chatty, confident little girl, though a bit of a tomboy, probably because of my three brothers. My Mary Quant doll was a tomboy, too. She came with a motorbike, dressed in a sleek catsuit, with bobbed red hair and was called Havoc. Depicted as a spy, she even had a parachute, she was extremely cool, and an equal to my brother's Action Man.

My brothers and I climbed trees, walls, and made dens. Thinking of this, the pea and strawberry heist comes to mind. It was a stealth operation which involved climbing over a six-foot wall, with one brother as a lookout, and stealing our grandparents' strawberries and peas mostly. We made a great gang of adventures, or so we thought.

Mention of climbing brings me to my point. Although I'm not a fan of heights, my middle brother has a much greater and somewhat irrational fear of heights. So, being the ever-helpful sister, I decided to fix it once and for all. Long story short, my brilliant plan to cure his fear involved demonstrating jumping off a roof.

My younger brother jumped off as instructed, but my middle brother refused — so I pushed him off. It wasn't very high, and I was only about nine, but I got into big trouble. In my mind, though, I was just trying to help him conquer his fear which, by the way, he still has. Sorry, Bro.

This story brings me to a memory of a CPD course I attended with a bunch of psychotherapists. Someone asked, "What if something I say or do makes a client's problem worse?" The facilitator replied, "As long as your intentions are good and kind, and you've followed professional guidelines, you'll do no harm."

Approaching any situation with care and good intentions are essential. Therapy doesn't have to be complicated; you could just start with a simple affirmation, breath practice, or maybe research some therapy online.

Many of our adventures took place over in the kissing ground adjacent to the old abbey. In the uneven fields covered in clover and dandelions, hours melted away as we were immersed in the quest for the elusive four-leaf clover. I had a desperate need to find one of those rare symbols of good luck, and eventually — with much determination and a little luck — I did. Dandelions with their delicate seeds became the next ritual, and with a big breath, the race to see whose seeds went the furthest and the highest. We'd often lie in the grass, looking up at the sky, creating wishes and dreaming dreams.

One year, the kissing ground played host to a small herd of cows, and the temptation to play cowboys was too great an opportunity to miss. After a fun afternoon herding the cows from corner to corner, the farmer appeared. A telling off, followed by a lecture on the potential dangers of these large animals, meant fantasy was abruptly replaced by reality.

The high walls of the old abbey stood as a formidable challenge to scale those ancient walls like modern-day explorers. The abbey, whispering tales of ancient times and ghost stories, added a mystical quality to the place. It's said that the spirits of long departed monks still lingered within the cloisters. Guardians of secrets buried beneath layers of the history of the abbey learned at school, daring one another to explore further. That brings me to the visualisation below.

VISUALISATION — DANDELION

Wish, Dream, Believe

Take a moment to close your eyes and imagine lying in a field on a sunny day, surrounded by vibrant yellow dandelions. The colour signifies the heat and power of the Manipura chakra, radiating warmth and energy. Take your awareness to your navel and feel the heat of Manipura.

Now pick a dandelion and watch it transform; petals turn to seeds. Inhale deeply, feel hope filling your lungs, and as you exhale, blow on the dandelion. Watch as the seeds disperse in all directions carried by the wind. Each seed represents a Wish, a Dream, a Desire, and Faith is the wind that carries them on their journey.

Now focus on one particular seed as it gracefully spirals down, and Trust in its ability to find fertile ground and germinate. Trust in nature's wisdom to see your Dreams take root and blossom. Then imagine a new crop of dandelions — each one a manifestation of your Wishes coming true; a field of bright yellow flowers, symbols of Hope.

Wishes are the flowering of Hope, but they must be carried by the winds of Faith and nurtured by the soil of Trust.

May your Wishes and Dreams come true.

Always Keep Dreaming.

WRITING A BOOK

You know, I've come to realise that being a writer doesn't mean you have to be some academic genius or a literary prodigy. And being a yoga teacher doesn't mean you have to fit into some mould of being super flexible, teetotal, or a strict vegan. It's funny how life works, because that little girl with those big dreams is the one who has something to share. I'm not someone who fits into those typical writer or yoga teacher stereotypes, and that's okay. In fact, it's more than okay; it's what makes me unique. I may not have a string of fancy titles, but I've got a story to tell, and I believe that all stories matter. You don't have to be famous; you don't have to have any qualifications; you just need to tell your unique story.

As for being a yoga teacher, yeah, I've been doing this now for a long time, and sure, I teach in a gym and in my own studio. Guess what! It's pretty great. I've had my fair share of raised eyebrows and judgmental comments: "Yoga in a gym?" "Oh, don't you teach in a studio?" Well, hello! Yoga isn't confined to some serene mountaintop or fancy expensive wellness retreat. It's for everyone, in all kinds of venues all over the world.

Teaching in a gym means I'm reaching people who might not have given yoga a try. It means I'm introducing this practice to people who may never step into a yoga studio. Isn't that what it's all about? Making yoga accessible? Unfortunately, this judgmental attitude about gyms is all too common. Who says yoga has to be practised in some mystical, spiritual place? Gyms are where people work on their health, their bodies, and their minds, and it's a place where they're already invested in their well-being, so why not bring more yoga to that space?

Seems so obvious to me, offering a practice that compliments their fitness routine. The point is: life isn't black and white. It's not about fitting into someone else's idea of what a writer/yoga teacher should be; it's about embracing who you are, sharing your experiences, and maybe inspiring someone else along the way.

So yeah, maybe I'm not a traditional writer or a stereotypical yoga teacher. There are plenty of those already, and I'm okay with that.

I read a quote somewhere that suggested the body of a bee aerodynamically isn't really designed to fly. Thinking of a Bumble Bee's large body and small wings, the quote continues with the statement that it's a good thing the bee doesn't know it's not built to fly. I really resonate with this, as I'm a little short, with strong but stocky legs, and unfortunately my physicality has prevented me from pursuing certain career paths. But it hasn't stopped me from trying most activities... which brings me to the Chinese fable about a frog. From memory, it goes something like this:

Hundreds of frogs faced the challenge of racing up a steep mountain, with the crowds chanting, "It can't be done; it's too steep and dangerous, you'll fall; it's impossible." One by one, the frogs fell, until there was only one left who managed to reach the top. Why did this frog succeed when hundreds failed? Well, the simple answer is that the frog that reached the top of the mountain was deaf and didn't hear the negative cries of the crowd below.

I don't always feel able to climb the mountain, and sometimes the negative voice is loudest. But through yoga, I always manage to find the right balance eventually, the wild Havoc adventurer balanced with the focused quiet moments of reflection and the never-ending pursuit of knowledge.

"I have no special talent, I am only passionately curious."

—Albert Einstein

DOGS

I've always had animals in my life, and from the age of six — after much cajoling (well begging, my dad) — we got our puppy, a cuddly ball of yellow naughtiness, and my family's love affair with dogs began.

As he grew, he proceeded to destroy everything in his path, with a particular fondness for shoes and my mum's slippers. Anyone that's seen the film *Marley and Me!* Will understand that was a carbon copy of our beloved pet labrador. His tail had the power to clear any coffee table and whip painfully across your legs, and he'd knock you over with his enthusiastic welcome and steal from any plate. I forgave him everything because he was my very best friend and my first real unconditional doggy love.

Just over twelve years later came the agonising decision at the vet's, unable to speak, only to nod in agreement. My best friend was suffering in pain, but still, I didn't want to say goodbye. I hugged him, taking in his familiar smell one last time, tears running down my face. It was the first of many grief-filled moments of loss, but life does go on, as they say. And although my first dog has never been forgotten, I've shared my life with many dogs since. And as I write this, the two chocolate labradors come to mind — such different characters, but my children's love for them parallel to my own.

We now have two Jack Russells — yes, I know, quite a difference from the labradors of old. Max, the larger of the two, was from a litter that Will's oldest friend had, and Dot joined us when he sadly passed away a few years ago — a brother and sister combo, I could write a whole book on the adventures of Max and Dot, but it would involve some scenes of horror, Jack Russells being notorious killers. Max in particular likes to eat everything in his path; Dot is a little too slow but I'm sure she was more than capable in her day.

You can tell where we've been walking because Max leaves a trail of holes along the way. His quest to dig up a mole has continued throughout his life, and yes, he has succeeded — only once, thankfully, as I wouldn't want to revisit that particular scene.

Max and Dot share with us the message of Santosha — Contentment and self-acceptance. Max, with his many missing teeth and tongue hanging out, and Dot, with her short, stumpy legs — neither focus on what they don't have. They're just happy as they are, living in the moment, without comparison or regret. It reminds us all that happiness comes from ourselves, not from comparing ourselves to others or longing for what we don't have, It's about appreciating what we do have and finding joy in the present moment.

So, a big thank you, Max and Dot, for reminding of me Santosha every day, with your simple, joyful existence.

YOGA ALL OVER THE WORLD

Vinyasa Flow — The art of linking movement and breath. It's something that transcends any school of yoga, a canvas open to our own interpretations, allowing us to integrate various styles into our practice. I've been fortunate enough to learn from an array of incredible teachers from studios all around the world, from workshops to retreats, one-to-one sessions to individual classes in India, and sessions in Hong Kong, Amsterdam, France, and Spain. Each experience has enriched my understanding, adding unique elements to my own practice and to my classes.

I remember a class in Hong Kong, led by a graceful Cantonese teacher who spoke no English. The studio was busy, and the lady at the desk explained that the class was in Cantonese. Undeterred, I thought we'd just hide at the back, but interestingly, most of the class was in Sanskrit and oddly familiar. I jotted down the routine in my journal, and the similarities to my practice weren't that surprising. After all, yoga is a universal practice.

That leads me to the point: yoga belongs to no one person, business, or company; it's not confined to a specific location, language, or style; you can practise wherever you like, however you like, on a sandy beach, in your cosy home, under the open sky in your garden, in a studio, one-to-one, or in a gym; you can choose to embrace it during an expensive retreat or during a simple session in your living room in front of a book, tv, or computer screen. The key is to practise and enjoy it with the freedom that suits you best. It's your choice. I know some exceptional teachers who I'd wholeheartedly recommend, but the beauty of yoga is that you have the liberty to find your own path.

That said, I've found that practising in a community setting offers its own array of benefits, mentally, physically, and emotionally. The camaraderie, the shared energy, and the guidance is an experience that can't be replicated alone. Sure, practising within a community comes at a cost, but there's a reason I teach at a gym, because I believe in making yoga accessible to everyone. In a gym, I can reach a wider group of people and I can, and do, break down stereotypes, proving that yoga is for everyone, everywhere. It's about embracing that spirit of inclusivity that makes yoga truly universal.

I remember joining the gym when it first opened — a space of opportunities and escape just waiting to be explored. The diverse classes and instructors provided a place where I could immerse myself in different forms of physical and mental well-being. And after my divorce it became a sanctuary, a safe place to go and simply be. When it was taken over, I began teaching, initially stepping in to cover classes for another instructor.

The studio's expansive space was both exciting and slightly intimidating, but little did I know it would become a canvas for some of my most enriching experiences in the years to come. Working at the gym connected me with an array of individuals, each with their own unique stories and aspirations. These people are more than just students. I was told once that befriending students wasn't professional, but who is to define what we should and shouldn't do? And looking back, I'm immensely grateful for the friendships that have blossomed from this shared journey. They have gifted me incredible moments, conversations, and connections that I wouldn't trade for anything.

Some of these remarkable souls have since departed from this world, leaving behind memories that hold a special place in my heart. Loss is a natural part of life, but it has been a reminder of the preciousness of every interaction, every shared experience, and that's the beauty of yoga. It's not just about the postures or the breath; it's about weaving connections.

I primarily teach Vinyasa flow (the synchronising of breath and movement), but it's important to clarify that I'm not confined by any specific yoga school. To me, yoga is a fusion of styles that I've learned from teachers and teachings across the globe.

In my classes, you'll witness this fusion, a collage of various techniques and styles that I've woven into my own unique offerings. I've had the privilege of learning from countless teachers, and my journey has led me to work with a diverse range of individuals, from young children to the wise and elderly, from busy business people to nurturing caregivers. I've taught across professions, cultures, and languages, all united under the umbrella of yoga.

For those who find it challenging to move to and from the floor, chair yoga is a wonderful option — a testament to the adaptability of yoga that we can find solace and empowerment from the seat of a chair. And let's not forget the deep restoration that Restorative and Yin classes bring. Here the pace slows, and we delve into stillness, letting the body and mind find their equilibrium.

So, here are a few glimpses into what I offer — a taste of my teaching. These classes reflect my experiences and are a testament to the ever-evolving nature of yoga.

Kneeling Sun Salutation

Moving from one pose to another is referred to as a vinyasa.

1. Sit back on the heels in an upright position (if this isn't possible, start from an upright kneeling position).
2. As you inhale, kneel up slowly and lift your arms to the ceiling.
3. Exhaling slowly, bring arms down to the floor and push buttocks back to the heels into extended child's pose.
4. Inhale forward onto your hands and knees, into cow pose.
5. Exhale into a downward-facing dog (lifting the knees and pushing back into the heels).
6. Inhale into a variation of upward facing dog, toes remaining curled under (dropping knees and hips towards the floor). Come to plank if upward facing dog is too challenging for your back.
7. Exhale, returning to downward facing dog.
8. Reverse the order of the vinyasa as you inhale, gently come onto your knees.

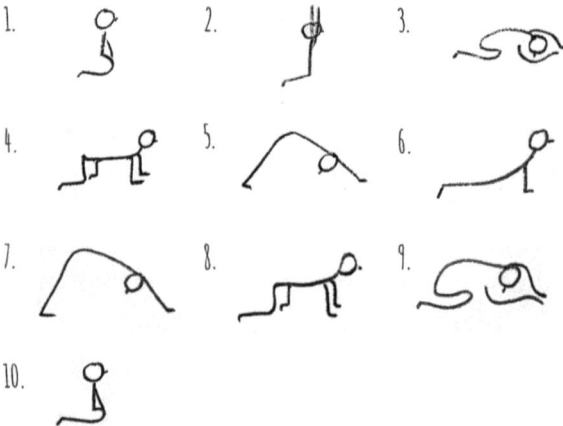

9. Exhale back into an extended child's pose.
10. Inhale and exhale into a seated position, sitting on the heels (if possible), and repeat the sequence four times or as many as you like.

I sometimes add cat, and tiger, to the sequence. Remember you can adapt any sequence to suit yourself.

Pause with eyes closed, now notice how you feel and take a few nice deep breaths.

YIN YOGA IN CYPRUS

I attended a relaxing, rejuvenating yin yoga class in Cyprus at Zening Resorts Latchi — a resort focusing on health and fitness with yoga and transformational breath-work, meditation classes, and no mobile phones or television. It called itself a quiet resort, with health and well-being as its intention, and certainly I found it a wonderful destination and visited several times.

A short walk down the steep hill took us into the little harbour, the buzz of restaurants, and a beautiful warm sea. Trips into the countryside were facilitated on quad bikes, and we enjoyed a visit and swim with the turtles in a protected bay which was magnificent. A visit to the Baths of Aphrodite was an absolute must, followed by snorkelling in the seas and caves nearby.

Unfortunately, I believe the resort is now closed, but I've continued to visit the area many times and still manage to find some yoga in Polis, which is just down the road.

Focusing on long holds, slow pace, and deep relaxation, Yin Yoga's emphasis is on holding passive stretches for longer periods of time, typically around 3-6 minutes. It targets the connective tissues to help release tension and increase flexibility and self-awareness.

YIN YOGA CLASS

Start seated with cross legs, if possible. Neck Rolls: turn head slowly from side to side, inhaling, slowly lift chin to the ceiling; exhaling, lower the chin to the chest, and hold (jalandhara bandha); release, lift chin, and repeat the sequence.

Lower onto the back. Bringing the soles of the feet together, knees fall apart, hold for 3-5 minutes (baddha konasana).

Slide both legs straight and flex toes to the ceiling. Engaging the legs, inhale, sliding the right heel along the floor towards the body, and exhale the knee out to the side. Hold for 1 minute, bring the knee back upright and slide the heel back along the floor, then repeat with the other leg.

With both legs extended, inhale the arms overhead, grab the left wrist and pull along the floor to the right; slide the right leg along the floor to the right, follow with the left leg, creating a banana shape, hold for 3 minutes. Repeat on the other side, bananasana.

Hug both knees into the body, apanasana, rock up to seated and over to hands and knees. Wide-leg child's pose, with head to one side then the other, curl toes under, and exhale to downward facing dog, then lower to the floor.

Seal pose — laying on the belly, take the hands to the corners of the mat and inhale to lift. Lift and lower until you find a comfortable height, then hold for 1 minute.

Come to child's pose, curl toes and lift knees to downward facing dog. Lift one leg and bring the knee to wrist, taking the opposite foot towards the other wrist, and lower to the floor in pigeon. Lower onto forearms and hold, then repeat on the other side.

Come to seated shoelace (gomukhasana). Either cross one leg over the other, bending the foot back, or the double leg version, knees on top of each other. Take one arm to ceiling and bend at elbow. Bringing palm of hand to the nape of the neck, and the other arm out to the side, bending towards the back and taking fingers to reach towards the other hand, grabbing the fingers in a bind. Hold and breathe 5 breaths each side.

Take the legs wide into straddle, place bolster or brick in front of the body, and forward fold, hold for 5 breaths. Bring legs together, placing bolster or bricks behind back in supported fish, hold for 3 minutes.

Come into constructive rest, feet to outer edges of the mat, knees rest against one another. Cover with a blanket and rest for 5-10 minutes.

INDIA WITH WILL, 2017

I had the pleasure of introducing my partner, Will, to the magic of this incredible country. It was a long-awaited trip, and I couldn't wait to see his reaction to everything India had to offer.

It started with a remarkable hotel, a true oasis of pure luxury and comfort after an arduous journey and never-ending queries at passport control, patience tested, yoga breathing engaged. It was paradise, and coincidentally my birthday, so a wonderful way to celebrate: India, holiday, yoga. The hotel staff were so lovely and surprised me with a cake and beautiful flowers in the room, and the infinity pool overlooking the countryside completed my wish list.

Stepping outside the hotel grounds, we were met with a different world, and the rural and raw beauty of India showed itself to Will in all its glory. Walking through paddy fields to the sea was a unique experience that immersed us in the local way of life, and I'll never forget the look of surprise on Will's face when the cows invaded the beach. He thoroughly enjoyed exploring all the local restaurants, loving the flavours, spices, and variety of rich Indian cuisine.

Despite all my efforts, I couldn't convince him to join me for the early morning yoga classes in the beautiful yoga shala overlooking the paddy fields, but it was ok. I wanted him to experience India in his own way and to find his unique personal connection, and he did. He embraced the traditional Ayurvedic treatments offered, finding his own sense of relaxation and rejuvenation.

This trip was a reminder of how different perspectives can enhance an experience, and for me witnessing India through Will's eyes added a new layer of appreciation and excitement. Sharing these precious moments and creating wonderful memories together was the most rewarding part of it all.

India has a way of staying with you long after you've left. It was a journey of discovery, relaxation, and growth; a journey that deepened our bond and left us with memories we'll treasure forever.

ONE OF THE YOGA CLASSES IN INDIA

Start seated with a mention of the importance of the breath and an explanation of what yoga is about, followed by three chants of Om. Coming then to stand in mountain, full forward fold, lifting back up and circling hips, side bend with arms to the ceiling. Standing tall, lift up onto toes, 3 repetitions, followed by side bends with hands clasped above the head. Forward fold with hands clasped behind back, then come to a steady jog progressing to lifting knees higher and higher. Take arms to one side, shoulder height, exhale fast across to the other side of your body, shouting 'ha' and repeat three times, then swap sides (gets rid of anger, stress, and frustration). Sun Salutation A with lunge, 4 repetitions. Sun Salutation B with warrior 1, warrior 2, warrior 3. Tree pose, onto floor Savasana for three minutes.

Cradle leg, repeat with other leg, rock up to boat and lower to the floor with one knee into the body. Lift the nose to knee and lower, swapping sides. Hug both knees into the body, rock up to seated butterfly, and fold forward. Come to kneeling cat, cow, tiger stretch, lower to floor locust, to bow, cobra, then come to seated lotus if possible. Alternate nostril breathing, followed by a meditation.

Being present in the moment, not forgetting the past lessons learned, excited about the future, but not dreaming of it.

Sankalpa — Intention for practice.

Ask yourself some questions:

What is your purpose? Perhaps bring that directly to your practice and ask: what do I want to achieve from this yoga practice?

YIN YOGA TRAINING

I had been looking for a Yin Yoga training course after I experienced the class in Cyprus. It resonated with me deeply, and I was eager to explore further the principles and techniques that yin yoga had to offer. Another teacher recommended a particular instructor and studio they believed would be the perfect fit for me.

I attended the four-day training, which included a stopover, and an opportunity to catch up with my oldest friend, enjoy a fabulous meal and evening discussing, well everything with a much missed friend.Through the following hours of practice, the study of philosophy, and benefits of yin poses, I realised how this practice would complement my existing teaching with its emphasis on long-held poses and deep stretches achieved slowly with mindful deep breathing. I felt a sense of connection and release that went beyond the muscular level through the excellent guidance of the yin teacher, and I began to unravel the layers of my practice and my own approach to teaching. I discovered that yin yoga was not just a series of postures; it was a philosophy that encouraged introspection, stillness, and acceptance.

Upon the completion of the course, I felt a renewed sense of purpose and excitement, and armed with a deeper understanding of yin yoga, I was ready to share it with my students, weaving yin postures into my classes. The transition from vinyasa flow sequences to the stillness of yin brought a sense of calm and introspection, the contrast allowing students to explore different dimensions of their practice, the active engagement of muscles, and the surrender of tension.

Introducing yin postures also opened up an avenue for me to guide my students towards a deeper connection with their bodies and breath. The longer holds in poses gave them the opportunity to listen to their bodies and observe their thoughts slowing down. I witnessed them embracing the quiet, meditative quality of yin, which contrasted beautifully with the yang energy of vinyasa flow. As they settled into the stretches, I encouraged them to explore sensations and emotions with acceptance.

Integrating yin postures offered a way to address the modern challenges of stress and overstimulation. In today's fast-paced world, we often neglect the importance of rest and introspection. But yin yoga provides a space to pause, disconnect, to cultivate patience. Incorporating yin postures into all my classes created a holistic feel and highlighted the point I keep making: yoga to yoke to join the union of strength and flexibility, effort and surrender, activity and rest, the balance of opposites that ultimately leads to harmony and growth. With each class, I witnessed my students leaving with a renewed sense of tranquillity and vitality. The integration of yin certainly added another layer of depth to their and my practice. It reaffirmed the power of a well-rounded practice.

As I continue to explore and share this practice with others, I am reminded that teaching is a journey of continued evolution. I continue to evolve as a teacher, constantly challenging and learning, embracing different styles and approaches with experience, and deciding what fits my teaching style whilst expanding my knowledge and understanding of yoga philosophy. The wisdom of ancient texts, like the Yoga Sutras and Bhagavad Gita, serves as a guiding light, offering insights that are as relevant today as they were centuries ago. This philosophical depth enriches my classes, infusing them with a sense of purpose and meaning far beyond the physical benefits. But it's an ongoing process, staying open to feedback and adapting my teaching to create an environment that supports my students. With each new insight, each exploration, I am reminded that the path of a yoga teacher is a journey of endless discovery.

"Your purpose in life is to find your purpose and give your whole heart and soul to it."

— Buddha

YOGAFIT IBIZA

Another retreat, but this time with my two dear friends who also happen to be yoga teachers. There were lots of different styles of yoga and many interesting talks, and always an opportunity to increase knowledge of yoga and deepen my practice.

These retreats are offered in April and October every year, situated on the coast of Ibiza overlooking the Mediterranean Sea and a beautiful sandy beach. The amazing thing about these retreats is the variety of classes and talks, from yoga to dance, fitness classes to meditation, candlelight yoga to sound baths, fitness pilates to Zumba, and much more, including talks on diet and nutrition, psychology, and mindfulness, etc.

Take a look at their website for the latest on what they have to offer.

I would definitely recommend this as a first retreat option due to the variety of talks and classes available.

SOLO RETREAT

Embarking on a solo retreat after lockdown. I was filled with a mixture of excitement and anticipation at the idea of immersing myself in a personal yoga practice. After lengthy research, I carefully selected a retreat that seemed promising.

However, as the experience unfolded, I found myself facing a mix of emotions, with a lingering hint of disappointment. The heart of any retreat is undoubtedly the teacher, the one who guides and inspires, but in this case the teacher did not quite meet my expectations. Their presentation lacked the engaging and knowledgeable qualities I was used to and had hoped for. Yet it's in moments like these that I am reminded of the wisdom shared by one of my first yoga teachers: "You learn something with every experience you have. It may not be what you wanted, but it has value." As I reflected on the retreat, even though it wasn't what I expected, I came to appreciate the valuable lessons that emerged.

This experience allowed me to reaffirm my comfort with solitude and the ability to relish a self-directed practice. It also reinforced the realisation that I have a wealth of yoga knowledge. So, rather than dwelling on disappointment, I've chosen to see it as an opportunity to learn that this retreat in its own way has strengthened my connection with my own practice, reaffirmed my ability to do things on my own, and find value in my own company. Igniting a renewed appreciation for the knowledge I've gathered throughout my yoga journey, it serves as a reminder that even in moments of disappointment, there is a silver lining of wisdom waiting to be uncovered.

"Life is like riding a bicycle, to keep your balance, you must keep moving."

—Albert Einstein

INTIMIDATION

Yoga, for all its qualities, can sometimes be accompanied by an air of intimidation. I recall an experience when I attended a class in London with a close friend, and while I won't mention the studio, the reception left much to be desired. The young woman at the initial reception seemed disinterested and unengaged, and it was tempting to slip into an employer mindset and ponder the need for customer service training. But I reminded myself to stay non-judgemental and simply focus on enjoying the yoga session.

In the changing room, the atmosphere was buzzing. I smiled and tried to make eye contact, but there was no response, and in the studio I received a few glances. Thankfully, my friend placed his mat next to mine, and I was relieved to see a friendly face.

I started to relax with his familiar energy next to me. The class began, led by a wonderful teacher who verbally guided us through a dynamic flow. The familiar asanas helped me relax, and although wheel is not my favourite go-to pose, I pushed up with ease. A genuine smile from another student during splits reassured me that perhaps the group was just initially wary of a newcomer.

As the class concluded, my friend and I rolled up our mats, then suddenly the group initiated a conversation with compliments about my practice, enquiries as to my background (lineage), and where I lived. It dawned on me that my proficiency in advanced poses had seemingly transformed me from an outsider to an accepted participant.

While I appreciated the kind words, I couldn't help but recognise the conditional nature of acceptance in this environment. Though the practice itself was enjoyable and invigorating, the realisation hit me that this was not the environment in which I wanted to practise yoga.

This experience is a reminder that yoga is about more than just physical prowess; it's about creating an inclusive and supportive community. My personal preference leans towards practising in an environment where kindness, acceptance, and genuine connection are the norm, where people are embraced for their unique journeys and not just their physical abilities. So, while that particular studio might suit those with a strong, confident practice, my practice thrives best in spaces where growth is nurtured and where yogis and yoginis can flourish together regardless of their skills.

A practice in Amsterdam evoked similar feelings. The teacher was aggressive and pushy, which led me to question myself. Was it my perception, or perhaps the way I was approaching these situations? But I realised through my various yoga classes, and years of experience, that energy and atmosphere can significantly impact the overall experience in any class. Sometimes, it's not about whether I'm in tune with the practice or not, but rather the compatibility between my energy and the environment I find myself in. Recognising what feels right and what doesn't is a valuable skill that allows me to seek out where I want to practise.

It's important to remember that the yoga journey is deeply personal, finding the places and practices that resonate with you. It's about acknowledging the dynamic interplay between our energy and the environment and allowing ourselves the freedom to seek spaces that nourish our souls and empower our individual practice. So, if you don't feel comfortable, if you're not enjoying the experience, if you don't like the teacher for whatever reason, walk away, or just don't go to that class again.

"No-one can make you feel inferior without your consent."
—Eleanor Roosevelt

RETREAT

Naughty moments when on retreat: It's almost like there's a magnetic force pulling me towards those rule-breaking moments. I've had my fair share of these rebellious episodes, always managing to find fellow mischief-makers in any group.

The memorable walk on the beach with a friend while the others were sleeping, ended with us both sharing drinks and a late night with the diving group in the hotel next door; the vodka-infused orange juice saga, three of us with mischievous grins, sipping our concoction, whilst sharing knowing glances and chuckles throughout the evening; the hunt for meat with a dear friend — while I dabble in the veggie life, he can't resist the call of a carnivorous feast and of course I've just got to go along for support. Then there's the forbidden red wine quest when another rebellious yogini and I ventured to a nearby pub, ignoring the retreat's ban on alcohol. The taste of that forbidden wine felt like a victory.

The memories of these naughty moments on retreat are a collection of shared secrets, laughter, and a touch of rebellion against the serenity of a yoga retreat. Although I'm not much of a drinker, it's the relentless Rules, Rules, Rules and society, with its ever-watchful eyes and wagging fingers, dictating to us that seems to drive me to naughtiness. After all, for some of us these retreats are an expensive treat, a break away from the stresses of everyday life, and therefore a time to relax and maybe enjoy the odd glass of wine or a meal of choice. Personally, I'm not that bothered by a ban on alcohol and meat, but it's just being told what I can and can't do that really gets my goat.

Moral of the story, you don't have to be a saint to go on a retreat. I can assure you, they really do want your business.

THE GAYATRI MANTRA

The Gayatri mantra, taken from the Rig Veda, is a sacred mantra. Deva Premal's rendition of this mantra beautifully captures its essence, evoking a deep spiritual connection. As you listen to her soothing voice, the powerful vibrations of the mantra resonate within, bringing a sense of tranquillity and inner harmony. It's a wonderful example of how sound and intention can be harnessed to uplift and inspire.

Om Bhur Bhuvah Svah

Tat Savitur Varenyam

Bhargo Devasya Dhimahi

Dhiyo Yo Nah Prachodayat

Translation

The absolute reality through the coming, going, and the balance of life. The essential nature illuminating existence is the adorable one, may all perceive through subtle intellect the brilliance of enlightenment.

This mantra's meaning goes beyond a simple translation. Here's a breakdown in more detail.

OM: This sacred syllable represents the divine, the source of all existence.

BHUR BHUVAH SVAH: These three words are known as the "Mahavyahrti" and represent the levels of existence. Bhur refers to the physical realm; Bhuvah to the mental or emotional realm; and Shah to the spiritual or celestial realm.

TAT SAVITUR VARENYAM: Tat refers to the ultimate reality beyond all three realms; Savitur refers to the divine sun or the source of all light and life; Varenyam means worthy of worship.

BHARGO DEVASYA DHIMAHI: Bhargo signifies the divine spiritual light that illuminates our understanding; Devasya refers to the divine reality; Dhimahi means meditate upon.

DHIYO YO NAH PRACHODAYAT: Dhiyo refers to our intellects or understanding; Yo means who; Nah means our; Prachodayat means inspire or guide.

The Gayatri Mantra is a calling for spiritual enlightenment and wisdom. It seeks the divine light to illuminate our minds and lead us from the darkness of ignorance to the clarity of understanding. The mantra is a prayer for guidance, wisdom, and higher consciousness, transcending the limitations of the physical, mental, and spiritual realms to connect with the ultimate reality. It is often chanted with devotion and a sincere intention to seek spiritual growth and realisation.

It's fascinating how slight variations of this mantra can lead to different subtle distinctions in its meaning.

I learned this from my teacher Steve, and he recorded a CD of him singing and playing the Gayatri Mantra. I've come to cherish this mantra, especially when in need of inspiration and a boost of healing. I lie down in a supported pose and just listen to its soothing melody. There's something incredibly peaceful and rejuvenating about it, restoring balance and equilibrium.

The multiple versions of this mantra show how universal its message is. It's like peering through different windows into the same serene landscape. Some translations emphasise the divine light, the sun, and our connection to the universe, while others highlight the transformative power it carries. But regardless of the specific translations, the essence remains a call for enlightenment, acknowledgement of ultimate reality, and divine guidance.

It's fascinating how a chant can hold such depth, providing a profound sense of peace, a tool to quieten the mind, and to find solace in the midst of life's chaos.

I found many motivational quotes and poems in my journals. Unfortunately, I can't find the original source of them all. There is one in particular by Erin Hanson (Australian poet) titled "Fall". Check it out. The internet is a valuable source of many inspirational quotes, so find the ones that relate to you. I tend to write them as notes in my journals to remind myself when in need of some extra motivation.

Consider the potential positive outcomes of taking risks and overcoming challenges. Instead of focusing on the fear of failure, shift to the possibilities of success. It's a reminder to embrace opportunities, step out of your comfort zone, and believe in the potential for achieving something great or even achieving something extraordinary. (I can hear my guru's reminder to embrace the teachings of yoga and become amazing.)

It reminds me of the story of the bird sitting on a branch. It is never afraid of the branch breaking, because its trust is not on the branch but in its own wings. (Unknown)

Always believe in yourself. Our true strength and resilience comes from within us. We should have faith in our own capabilities and trusting our abilities to navigate through life's challenges, encouraging self-confidence and resilience.

"'Come to the edge,' he said. They said, 'We are afraid.'

'Come to the edge,' he said. They came. He pushed them, and they flew."

— Guillaume Apollinaire

MINDFULNESS

Mindfulness is the practice of being fully present in the current moment, cultivating a deep awareness of whatever is happening around and within you. Mindfulness encourages us to engage with the world without being preoccupied with regrets about the past or worries about the future. It's about giving our complete attention to what's happening now at this moment, whether it is practising yoga, driving, or engaging in a conversation. When we practise mindfulness, we consciously focus on one thing at a time, allowing any distractions to be placed in the background, engaging on our immediate experience. In doing so we open ourselves up to a heightened sense of awareness and a richer connection to our surroundings.

This practice helps to manage stress, anxiety, and overwhelming thoughts. It helps tone down the noise in our heads, the constant chatter of the monkey mind.

I repeat the mantra from earlier in the book — Yogash Chitta Vritti Nirodhah, which is a Sanskrit phrase from Patanjalis yoga sutras, often translated as "yoga is the cessation of the fluctuations of the mind". Calming the mind's constant chatter and restlessness through various practices and disciplines, the sutra portrays the idea that yoga is not merely a physical practice but a holistic system integrating the mind, body, and spirit with a view to finding connection, balance, and harmony.

Stress can manifest itself in various ways throughout our bodies, affecting our physical, mental, and emotional well-being, muscle tension, headaches, digestive issues, stomach ache, constipation, nausea, immune system issues, making you more susceptible to illness and infections, cardiovascular effects such as blood pressure irregularities, hypertension, respiratory shallow breathing, skin conditions, sleep disruptions, interfering with sleep patterns, cognitive effects, difficulties in concentration, memory function, decision-making, emotional symptoms, mood swings, irritability, anxiety, depression, weight fluctuations due to changes in appetite, hormonal imbalances, and hair loss.

It's important to note that individuals can and do indeed experience stress differently, based on genetics, overall health, coping mechanisms, and individual circumstances. Managing stress effectively through relaxation techniques, mindfulness exercise, healthy eating, social support, and seeking professional help when needed, can help mitigate its negative impact on the body and mind.

Here are some ideas, relaxation tips, and sample breathing exercises:

Practise self-care by dedicating some time each day to activities that bring you joy and relaxation, whether it's reading, going for a walk, or even having a soak in the bath. None of these activities are expensive.

Listen to music or mantra.

Mindful breathing: taking time throughout the day to focus on your breath, inhaling deeply through the nose, exhaling through the mouth 5 times, letting go of tension.

Follow yoga breathing exercises.

Limit your screen time, both phone, computer, and TV.

Limit time spent with negative people.

Stay hydrated, drinking plenty of water throughout the day.

Connect with nature and spend time outdoors, as nature has a calming effect on the mind. Take your shoes off and connect directly with the earth.

Practice gratitude by keeping a journal and writing down things you're grateful for every day.

Stay active with regular physical activities such as yoga, walking, cycling, swimming, running — whatever works to boost your mood.

SPAs — most spas and gyms offer yoga classes. I've attended some great classes at a local day spa. They have a wide selection of classes:

Yoga flow, HIIT yoga, Slow Yin yoga, Fitness Pilates, Hatha yoga, Stretch and Relax, Meditation, Restorative yoga, and Sound Healing sessions.

There's something for everyone to try.

BREATHING EXERCISES

Bhramari

Humming Bee Breath Pranayama. This breath is a beneficial technique in yoga that offers numerous advantages, including its impact on vocal quality and focus.

How to practise Bhramari Pranayama:

First, find a comfortable seated position, spine straight and shoulders relaxed. Close your eyes and bring your attention to your breath. Inhale deeply and exhale completely for three calming breaths. Now, use your fingers and thumbs to close your ears and eyes. Take a deep breath through the nose; as you exhale, create a humming sound, like that of a bee, and continue to exhale the humming sound for the complete duration of the exhalation. Continue this process for several rounds, focusing on the vibrating sound.

Benefits of Bhramari Pranyama:

Calming effect: The humming sound and the gentle vibration created during Bhramari Pranyama have a soothing effect on the nervous system, helping to reduce stress and anxiety.

Voice Quality Improvement: Regular practice of Bhramari Pranayama is believed to help improve the quality of your voice, making it clearer, which is why it's great for teachers, public speakers, and performers.

Focus and Concentration: The focus on the humming sound and the rhythmic breathing pattern helps to calm the mind and enhance concentration.

Relief from Tension: The vibrations of the humming sound can help release tension in the facial muscles, which can help relieve headaches.

Energy Balance: This pranayama helps balance the energy channels in the body and can be especially useful when you're feeling mentally fatigued.

Rhythmic Breathing

This practice requires control of the breath by counting the inhalation, retention, exhalation, and relaxation of the breath.

For example:

INHALE THE BREATH, count to 6; RETAIN THE BREATH, count to 3

EXHALE THE BREATH, count to 6; PAUSE THE BREATH, count to 3

You can increase the count, remembering to keep the inhalation the same as the exhalation and the retention the same as the relaxation. And you can repeat as many times as you want. This method allows the mind to focus on counting, guiding awareness to the breath.

Square Breathing

This method is similar to Rhythmic Breathing:

INHALE THE BREATH, count 6; RETAIN THE BREATH, count 6

EXHALE THE BREATH, count 6; PAUSE THE BREATH, count 6

Remember to breathe through the nose. This method of breathing is extremely relaxing. Remember this is just a guide and you can count for longer and repeat as many repetitions as you need. Just notice how you feel. All of these breath practices can be found on the internet.

NB: Do not practise breath retention if pregnant.

MY LOVE OF BOOKS

My love of books was ignited at a young age as I disappeared into the pages of many great stories. My shelves were adorned with titles such as *Stig of the Dump*, the captivating Black Beauty series, the mysterious allure of Nancy Drew and The Hardy Boys, the Famous Five, heartwarming *Little Women*, and the insightful tales of James Herriot. I lost myself in vibrant adventures and distant landscapes, and each story not only entertained me but also served as a guiding light, sparking my curiosity and fuelling my interests. As I turned the pages, these books became more than just stories. They were gateways to new realms of understanding and imagination, shaping the person I am today.

A journey through my home now and the presence of books is still obvious, an array of genres inviting exploration and discovery. Fiction tales breathe life into imaginary worlds, biographies open windows to remarkable lives, while non-fiction works beckon with wisdom and facts. A journey through my home is a journey from yoga, meditation, to the vibrant allure of photography and travel, gardening, a bit of cooking and design, and the breadth of my passions. Anatomy and psychology books stand side by side, encouraging a deeper understanding of the human mind and body. Hypnotherapy and philosophy engage my thoughts, and references await my enquiries. Every book is a treasure trove of insight waiting to be unearthed and shared. A perfect day for me begins and ends with a book.

It is never too late to pick up a book and start reading. There's really no excuse not to read, with local libraries in every town, audiobooks, eBooks, charity shops, and of course, let's not forget our fabulous local book shops, which offer amazing choices, expert advice, and sometimes tea and cake.

Book Shops

Some of the fabulous independent book shops I've had the pleasure of visiting while travelling around in the camper.

*   High Peak Bookstore & café, Ashbourne Road, Buxton.
*   Barter Books, Alnwick Station, Northumberland.
*   The Bookshop, Main Street, Wigtown, Scotland.
*   Bookmark, The Crescent, Spalding, Lincolnshire.
*   The Brazen Head Bookshop & Gallery, Burnham Market, Norfolk.
*   Leakey's bookshop, Church Street, Inverness, Scotland (recommended by my fabulous niece)
*   My go-to books are listed at the end.

PAIN

I woke one morning in the most horrendous pain, barely able to move and clutching my abdomen. It was akin to labour pains, coming like waves across my lower abdomen and back. Long story short, kidney stones were diagnosed by the doctor, along with the comment, "Goodness me, you are in a lot of pain." *Somewhat of an understatement*, I thought at the time.

She gave me a prescription for some strong painkillers, but the subsequent scan revealed a tumour in my left kidney. Then followed the six months of monitoring and more CAT scans.

The recent road trip across Europe to the Italian Lakes on the motorbikes became a distant memory. Just as everything in life had been going so well – back on the motorbike, successfully teaching, and helping people through Hypnotherapy/Psychotherapy, just selling my house and moving forward again, the exciting prospect of a yoga studio of my own, and the new cottage shared with my partner. It was with a heavy heart, some tears, and sadness, that I contemplated my wish to do so much more with my life. Please let me be ok.

I got out the yoga reference books and I practised mantra, mudras, breath-work, restorative and yin yoga. I meditated, and thankfully, six months later, the tumour had magically dispersed. (When asked the urologist said it's just one of those unexplained medical mysteries).

The word tumour had sent me into a panic, and although this had been a stressful time, I realised again that this was a stark reminder: Live life, live every moment fully. We do not know what the future holds for us before we take that last breath.

That brings me back to the Bhagavad Gita, my copy tatty and well-thumbed. Each time I read it, I'm blessed with an inner strength that sees me through the challenges I face.

Find a book, a quote, a poem, a podcast, an affirmation, something to inspire you, to encourage you, to find that all-important inner strength to see you through the extremely challenging and tough times.

While I don't hold any medical qualifications or the title of grief counsellor, my life's journey has gifted me a mass of experiences. I've navigated the agony of numerous injuries and surgeries; I've intimately known the ache of bidding farewell to dear friends and loved ones, holding hands and witnessing their last breath; I've journeyed through the labyrinth of postnatal lows, emerging stronger; I've made my fair share of missteps, learning from each one; I've cherished and let go; I've tasted both success and failure. And from these experiences I've cultivated resilience.

I've amassed a toolkit of practical insights garnered from these encounters with life's trials. My journey through education has been as diverse as my life and includes a multifaceted range of subjects, from Business Studies and Social Studies to Psychology, Yoga, Hypnotherapy, Psychotherapy, Sports Massage, Aromatherapy, Typing and Office Practice, Accounts, and Beauty Therapy. I even hold a motorcycle MOT manager qualification.

And while much of this is seemingly unrelated to the realm of yoga and holistic practices, it's a testament to a life filled with surprises. These qualifications are not just pieces of paper. They are the milestones that make a dedication to learning and personal growth, each area of study equipping me with a versatile skillset to connect with and serve others in various capacities.

The point is, I believe it's never too late to pick up a book, to take a course, or to try something new. It's tough sometimes, though. I admit I'm presently struggling with an online photography course, which is totally out of my comfort zone and involves dealing with technology, which is definitely not my forte. But I love it, and as a result decided to join an evening photography course at my local college. I've just completed it and have learned so much from my lovely tutor, who was again another fortunate find.

"Intelligence is the ability to adapt to change."
—Stephen Hawking

That brings me back to Motorbikes: from a Motorcycle Dealership to a yoga sanctuary.

Becoming a Company Secretary and Financial Director of a motorcycle dealership was never part of my grand plan. I didn't particularly aspire to be an employer, and I certainly didn't dream of shouldering the responsibilities of health and safety. Managing a business in a windowless office, poring over accounts, and wrestling with invoices felt like a far cry from the life I had envisioned.

I could fill pages with tales of my experiences in that world, but the truth is I have no desire to return to that dark room, where the light came from a fluorescent tube and a flickering computer screen, and where cash flow was my constant companion. It was a chapter of my life that I had to navigate, but it wasn't where my heart truly belonged. However, life has a way of surprising us when we least expect it.

After my divorce, the business underwent a transformation, moving and expanding onto a new industrial estate, and it was there amongst this unexpected journey that I received a visit from the owner of a new yoga studio situated on the same estate. Introducing herself, our mutual love of yoga was discussed and what followed were regular visits to support her fledgling studio and, more importantly, to continue my yoga practice.

Jivamukti yoga became my sanctuary, my refuge from the demands of the corporate world, a stark contrast to my office days, a space filled with warmth, light, and the gentle guidance of yoga instructors. Those classes became the highlights of my working days, moments of respite and renewal that made the challenges of the business world more manageable.

I'm pleased to say that after all these years, the studio is still open on that industrial estate, serving as a beacon of light and serenity amid the hustle and bustle of business life. It's a testament to the power of yoga to transform not just individuals but also the spaces and communities it touches.

NAVIGATING THE UPS AND DOWNS OF BUSINESS OWNERSHIP

Running a business brings with it quite a few challenges, and one of the most trying can be dealing with problematic employees. Everyone seems to know how to do your job better than you, yet they don't want to step up and take the risks themselves. Instead, they choose to critique and criticise. I know the frustration of facing such problematic employees who seem more interested in finding faults than finding solutions. I've walked that treacherous path where the boundaries between professional disagreements and personal attacks blurred into a disconcerting haze. Nothing can truly prepare you for the shock and disappointment of discovering someone you entrusted has resorted to deception and betrayal. It's a stress-inducing process; one that can leave you feeling drained and disheartened.

I vividly remember the day I found myself in the middle of an unpleasant tribunal. I made the decision to represent the company myself. It was a gamble to weigh the costs and benefits of pursuing what was fair and just, but fire and outrage burned. I knew that standing up for what was right, even in the face of a daunting challenge, was a principle worth fighting for.

So, I rolled up my sleeves, and an employee and I dove headfirst into the intricacies of representing the company in the tribunal. Unfortunately, I'd just had surgery on my knee and was still on crutches, but the judge kindly allowed me to remain seated throughout the proceedings. It was a steep learning curve, one that demanded time, energy, and resilience. But it was also a transformative experience, and one that reinforced my commitment to justice and my belief in the power of perseverance. I needed to stay calm, so yoga to the rescue again. A few rounds of alternate nostril breathing, followed by slow regular breaths, helped me stay calm and collected throughout the proceedings.

There's a certain satisfaction that comes from uncovering the truth, from finding the evidence that exposes a lie. It is a triumph of integrity over dishonesty, a reminder that even in the face of deceit, the truth eventually prevails. Even many years later, there are many stories that emerge from the betrayals I've encountered throughout my life. But with a commitment to upholding the values that define who we are and what we believe, even in the darkest moments the light of truth can shine through illuminating the path forward.

The Sanskrit word Satya means Truthfulness — honesty. It teaches us to be honest with ourselves, to confront our own truths, and to live authentically; a call to embrace the truth.

I practise Satya in my life and as a theme for class, first discussing the meaning, then how we can bring truthfulness into the practice of yoga.

"The most dangerous person is the one who listens, thinks, and observes."
— Bruce Lee

ROAD TO RESILIENCE

Travelling back from visiting friends in Norfolk — a fabulous afternoon spent in their garden overlooking the lake — I was on the back of my partner's Hayabusa (motorbike). We stopped at a busy roundabout junction, and the car behind us collided with the bike, sending me hurtling through the air, landing unceremoniously on the car's bonnet then rolling onto the busy road.

My partner amazingly managed to hold onto the handlebars after losing his grip, regained control, and averted what would have been a catastrophic crash. Dazed and disoriented, I crawled to the safety of the verge, fumbling with my gloves, trying to undo the helmet strap that felt tight around my neck.

The driver of the car kept insisting I keep the helmet on, but my partner stepped in to defend my right to breathe and helped me free myself from the constricting helmet. Once it was off, I focused on the rhythm of my breath and slowed it down, finding calmness in the chaos of traffic and onlookers, and I started to feel calmer. What felt like minutes later, the ambulance arrived. The paramedic checked my vital signs, blood pressure, and pulse, wore an expression of astonishment that they were all inexplicably normal, defying the odds of such a traumatic incident.

"That's her yoga breathing," my partner explained, and I couldn't help but smile through the residual shock. Amid the chaos, a policeman poked his head around the door of the ambulance, seeking a statement for what he believed was a clear case of dangerous driving. I, however, disagreed and refused to cast blame. It was an accident and should be labelled as such. That in itself had been trauma enough for the driver of the car.

It was my son's 21st birthday party, and my determination to be there propelled me forward. I couldn't miss this significant occasion. So, despite the advice of the paramedic who wanted to take me to hospital, I climbed back on the motorbike and headed home. The journey felt like an endurance test, every bump and jolt reminding me of the moments earlier. As the evening arrived, I relied on a combination of painkillers and a few glasses of wine to keep the discomfort at bay. Not going to the celebration wasn't even a consideration. I had made a promise to be there, and I intended to keep it.

The night was filled with laughter, a fun night spent celebrating this milestone birthday.

However, the following day was a stark reminder of the toll such resilience can take and the need for rest, recovery, and finding that all-important balance. The mix of painkillers and alcohol left me feeling battered, bruised, and unwell. The party had been worth it, but my body was making sure I knew the cost.

A mother's determination, with a bit of yogic strength, a journey from crash to celebration, a testament to the power of love and commitment. It's a reminder that sometimes the pain and discomfort we endure are small prices to pay for the moments of joy and connection that make life truly meaningful.

"You're braver than you believe, stronger than you seem, and smarter than you think."

—AA Milne

HOT YOGA

Venturing into the world of Bikram yoga was an intriguing experience that left me both amazed and slightly bewildered. The 26 poses performed at 40c for 90 minutes took me by surprise, especially the lack of breathable air and the torrents of sweat that seemed to pour from every pore. It was then that I understood the necessity of placing a towel on the mat — an ingenious technique to maintain grip and composure.

The instructor's approach was engaging and dynamic, delivering instructions without demonstrations but with humour and a fierce energy. She led us through the sequences, coaxing and encouraging us to push our boundaries. As I attempted to maintain my balance in poses like Padangusthasana (big toe grab), I grappled with the challenge of gripping my slippery toes, a task made even more daunting by the relentless heat. I found myself needing to pause and catch my breath, my heart pounding like a drum in my chest, while the instructor (a fabulous teacher who I ended up going to India with) persistently urged me to "get up" while grinning, only adding to the intensity.

Post-class, my skin felt rejuvenated, and I experienced an invigorating buzz throughout my body. I couldn't help but reflect on the elevated heart rate and its potential implications for individuals with certain health conditions. In essence, I walked away from this hot yoga adventure recognising its potential benefits, particularly in terms of detoxification and the sense of exhilaration it provided.

My Bikram experience taught me to approach every style of yoga with an open mind and to respect the individual needs of our bodies.

LOSS

The year 2021-2022 was marked by a series of losses that left my partner and me reeling, the departure of dear friends and family leaving behind an emotional whirlwind.

One particular night remains etched in my memory. As we walked out of the hospital, the realisation that we wouldn't see or speak to my stepfather again left me engulfed in a sea of sorrow, especially for my dear mother. He passed away one-and-a-half hours before my class at the gym. Fatigue clung to me like a shadow, having spent most of the night grappling with my emotions.

The idea of cancelling the class crossed my mind, but it felt too late for that, so with a heavy heart and weary eyes, I gathered myself, steadied my breath, and focused instead on my students that morning. Once the class started, I found myself moving to the rhythm of the class, and for those moments I was able to anchor myself to the present. The pain and sorrow were still there, but they shared space with a sense of purpose and connection. It wasn't easy, and there were moments when my voice wavered, but I found sanctuary in the practice. It was a reminder that life continues even in the face of loss.

It reinforced the lesson that while grief can be overwhelming, there are threads of strength woven through our experiences that help us navigate the storm, and a poignant reminder that life must go on. I found a little balance and peace amongst the turmoil. And in that moment, I understood the power of my yoga practice, not just as a physical discipline but as a tool to carry us through the most challenging aspects of life.

Bhagavad Gita — Accept the knocks of life as blessings in disguise, and be unaffected by the bad or good things that happen to you.

"He who binds himself to a joy doth the winged life destroy, He who kisses the joy as it flies, lives in eternities Sunrise."

—William Blake

LOCKDOWN, ZOOM, AND CHARITY

During lockdown, I decided to start conducting yoga classes through Zoom. It was an unexpected twist in my yoga career and a way to adapt to the circumstances. The virtual classes turned out to be a lifeline for many, offering relief and support during unprecedented and challenging times. These sessions brought people together on their screens, providing unity and community. Although never a replacement for in person live classes, it was nevertheless a reminder of how yoga can help navigate even the most uncertain times. Depending on your budget and experience, YouTube has lots of free yoga classes, and you can even follow your favourite teacher online wherever you are in the world with an internet connection.

I wasn't actively teaching at the gym, but I was still being paid and earning online, so I continued to donate to the food bank. I've been supporting various charities throughout my adult life, as I've always believed in giving back when I can.

I've been fortunate to have the support of my family when I needed it most. Yes, I've been skint, and it was a miserable time in my life when everything was hard and a struggle. It really made me think, what would we have done without our family's food and clothes parcels? What happens to people who don't have that kind of family support?

I've received some incredibly generous contributions over the years from friends and students. Thank you for filling up my car with chocolates for the kids at Christmas, tea, coffee, biscuits, and everyday essentials for the rest of the year.

LOCKDOWN ZOOM CLASS

Start seated. Focus for the practice — Non-Harming — Ahimsa. Mantra: "Today I will practise Kindness."

"This week I will be kind to myself, family and friends. I will be kind to all I come into contact with."

Breathe in the intention and continue to practise this intention all week.

Inhale, breathing only through the nose, and exhale to an easy twist; inhale back to centre and repeat. Inhale, lifting the right arm to the ceiling, and exhale, reaching the arm to the left. Repeat on the other side. Inhale, arms to the ceiling, and exhale to a forward fold. Grabbing the feet, swap cross of legs, and repeat the sequence.

Come onto back, inhale, knees into chest, exhale to hug knees.

Easy Bridge — with feet placed onto the floor, hip distance apart, inhale, lifting the arms and hips (with a block/brick in-between knees), exhale arms to the floor behind head and squeeze the block/brick, inhale to pause then exhale hips down, inhale and repeat the sequence 5 times.

Inhale, knees into body, and exhale as you hug knees — apanasana. Inhale, extending both legs to the ceiling; exhale, lifting body up, and reach opposite hand to the outside edge of the knee, whilst allowing the other leg to drop and hover off the floor. Inhale, back to centre before repeating opposite leg; 5 repetitions each leg.

Reclined happy baby — inhale, taking hold of the outside of the feet; exhale, pull the bent knees towards armpits, rock from side to side. Inhale, then exhale to straddle legs (taking legs wide), inhale return to happy baby, exhale straddle legs. Inhale happy baby, bending knees towards armpits and holding feet, exhale straddle legs, inhale happy baby.

Rock up and down, rock up and over to hands and knees (or just come to hands and knees). This is when I use my kneeling pad, placed under my knees for extra padding.

Exhale to extended child's pose (pushing buttocks to heels). Take hands together, resting on elbows, inhale lifting hands together in prayer; exhale, bring hands back to the floor, shoulder width apart; inhale, lift knees 2 inches off the floor and hold for 5 seconds; exhale, straighten both legs, downward facing dog. Inhale, lower the knees 2 inches off the floor, hold for 5 seconds; exhale, straighten legs to downward facing dog; exhale stepping to a forward fold, inhale to standing, mountain, sun salutation A. Inhale, flow to lunge, and repeat flow to exhale lunge twist; repeat on the other side. Sun salutation B with warrior 123, extending one leg to standing split. Repeat on the other side.

Flow to lizard (step one foot to the outside edge of the wrist, dropping the back knee to the floor, allow the front of the body to lower, coming onto forearms or brick). Moving with the flow of your breath, step back and lift into plank, with the knees off the floor to side plank, coming onto the side of the body with only the foot and hand on the floor. Repeat each side. Optional advanced hanumanasana sequence, splits.

Standing balance, dancers, natarajasana — focus the gaze on a point in front of you, inhale and grab one foot behind, bent at the knee, and exhale pushing the foot into the hand, extending the leg behind. Extend the opposite arm at the same time. Repeat on the other side.

Childs pose for 5 breaths, step to plank, and lower to the floor.

Inhale, lifting to half bow/full bow. (Half bow, lying on the front of the body, bring forearms to the floor, push into sphinx, bend one knee and reach back for the foot, push foot away, and push into opposite forearm or hand. Grab feet with both hands for full bow.)

Child's pose for a few breaths, push up to kneeling, and come to seated.

Gomukhasana (cow face). Seated shoelace, cross legs, knees on top of one another, calves and ankles pulled back on the floor against thighs (stretching the front of the foot and ankle). Arms either stretched to ceiling, with hand bent back to the nape of the neck stretching the tricep, or grabbing the hand with the opposite hand. Release the arms/hands and uncross the legs, lean back and swap sides. Come onto back and repeat happy baby to straddle. Notice how it feels different each side. Don't forget to breathe.

Easy twist with knees together, moving from side to side with the breath; inhale, hold one side, bringing palms together in a closed twist to exhale, open twist, 3 repetitions.

Savasana or Constructive Rest with knees bent feet apart, 10 minutes relaxation.

Visualise the body sinking into the floor, becoming heavier and heavier with every exhalation, relaxing more and more with each breath. Start to count the inhales and see if you can make the exhales a little longer. Continue for 5 complete breaths.

Continue to rest or come back to seated.

MENOPAUSE

The M word — as I nicknamed it — is all around me. I used to think it wouldn't happen to me, that I'd gracefully — well, maybe not gracefully — bypass all the symptoms my friends complained about, like night sweats, day sweats, memory loss, brain fog, achy painful joints, low libido, disrupted sleep, and itchy skin. But menopause hit me, waking me one night with a puddle on my chest and some confusion as to why my sheets were wet.

I couldn't remember dates, times, and conversations, my joints creaked and ached like my old staircase, and my once vibrant libido had gone into hiding. Even my skin itched incessantly. I started to forget simple words, the kind of words that had once been on the tip of my tongue. It was as if my vocabulary had been scattered to the wind, leaving me grasping for phrases that used to flow effortlessly.

Teaching became a battle, as my mind played tricks on me, going blank mid-sentence time and time again. I would stand there, staring at my students, my heart racing, confidence slipping through my fingers like sand. I had to refer back to my notes, those precious lifelines, to find my way back to the session I'd planned. Frustration welled up inside me, and with each forgotten word, each awkward pause, my self-confidence took a beating.

I soldiered on, though, determined not to let this phase of life define me. But there were days when I wondered if I should throw in the towel and give up teaching. I felt stupid and useless, a shadow of my former self. I was tired, physically, mentally drained, and emotional. As the mirror reflected a face with no sparkle, it was as if I had simply lost my mojo. That vibrant energy that used to radiate from within had long gone. Menopause had wrapped its arms around me, but deep down, I knew it would pass. I couldn't let this phase of my life defeat me, I'd been through so much.

So, I embarked on a quest to reclaim my memory, confidence, vitality, and mojo. With the help, support, and advice of trusted friends, and of course, a regular yoga practice — albeit a slower and more gentle self-practice — I began to feel more like my old self. My friends were the compass pointing me in the right direction, always there and open about their own experiences, happy to listen and share what worked for them. They reminded me that forgetfulness and fatigue were not signs of weakness but moments in life that would pass.

The healing power of yoga slowly started to work its magic, nurturing and guiding me back to a place of balance and self-assuredness. Through this practice, I reconnected with my body and mind, coming to a place of acceptance. I learned to listen to new-found wisdom, an inward rediscovery of my own strength and resilience, finding my inner adventurer again — the adventurer who wasn't afraid to embrace change, who saw each new day as an opportunity to grow, and who believed that life's challenges were just stepping stones to greater wisdom and self-love.

There is a way through this maze of menopause. The adventure of life is never truly over. It just takes on new and exciting forms.

REVIVING THE RIDER WITHIN ME

After the accident in October 2008, I couldn't imagine ever riding again. The memory of that fateful night loomed large in my mind, casting a shadow over the joy I had once found on two wheels. My Honda sat neglected in the garage, collecting dust, a silent testament to a passion I had once enjoyed. Years passed, and the motorcycle remained a relic of days gone by; I had resigned myself to the idea that the thrill of the open road was no longer for me.

One day, totally out of the blue, someone asked a simple question: "Why don't you ride it any more?" And as those words hung in the air, I wondered, why not indeed? I could see the mixture of anticipation and concern on my partner's face, as he had been trying to quietly but persistently urge me to take up riding again, and my response carried the weight of years of hesitation and uncertainty.

My partner's support had been unwavering, his encouragement a gentle nudge toward reclaiming a part of myself I'd tucked away. Sometimes, the greatest gift we can give each other is the space to heal and the freedom to rediscover the things that bring us joy. After the accident, I had lost my confidence, the belief in my own abilities that had once propelled me towards the open road with a smile on my face.

The day after that pivotal conversation, the old Honda roared back to life, ready for its new MOT and the promise of new adventures. And with a renewed sense of confidence, I swung my leg over the bike, feeling the familiar weight and power beneath me. It was a moment of exhilaration, a return to something that had once brought me so much pleasure. My passion reignited, and with my partner's encouragement, I embarked on a new chapter of riding. It was a testament to the transformative power of support and belief, and a reminder that sometimes all it takes is someone who sees your potential and encourages you to believe in yourself.

After reigniting my passion, I decided to take a bold step forward and I purchased a new Ducati Monster — a symbol of both power and elegance. The confidence in my new bike was like a shot of adrenaline. With the sleek lines of the Ducati beneath me and the wind rushing past, I embarked on my first long journey alone. It was a solo adventure that was in equal parts exciting and liberating. Each twist of the throttle felt like a reclaiming of my independence and a reaffirmation of my spirit. As the miles stretched out before me, I revelled in the feeling of being on the open road, free to explore, free to be myself.

This desire to ride more led me to the yoga weekend with Steve, my guru. It was an achievement that held deep personal meaning. Riding alone to Sheffield, I had come full circle, and it felt like a triumph. With the rumble of the Ducati beneath me and the promise of adventure, both my passions united in one weekend.

Riding in the shadows:

confronting ghosts with yoga breath, life has a way of reminding us that even as we move forward, the ghosts of our past can still cast their shadows.

In the company of friends on a ride out that should have been exhilarating, I found myself confronted by a fear of riding at night, the shadows from the moon playing tricks. As the panic took hold, I dropped behind and finally pulled over. The realisation washed over me that I wasn't ready to face the challenge of riding at night. It was a humbling moment, a stark reminder that healing and recovery are journeys marked by both progress and setbacks.

I refused to be defeated by fear, though. Instead, I turned to the practice that had been my solace throughout this journey — yoga breathing. I took my helmet off and started to count my breath, now with a steady rhythm, and the panic slowly subsided.

Now when I ride at night, you'll catch me chanting mantras and concentrating on my breathing (with open eyes and focusing on the road, of course).

It's a reminder that we all have our battles, our ghosts, and our moments of vulnerability, but with the power of breath and the strength of determination, we can face even the darkest of shadows and emerge on the other side, strong and more resilient than before, embracing vulnerability, confronting fears, and finding the courage to ride through the night, both on the road and in the depths of our own minds.

Talking of Trauma:

do you remember what you were doing on 9/11? My memory of that day at Cadwell Park.

Racing Legends and Track Day Thrills. Amongst the roar of motorbike engines and the exhilaration of track days, our venture into the world of motorsports as a Suzuki dealership was the result of a decision to sponsor racing and introduce track days. It was very much my partner's idea, so after some number crunching the company proceeded to organise some track days at Cadwell Park race track. And with the help of guest riders, racing icons, up-and-coming, now famous successful racers, the journey into racing and track days began. In amongst the roaring engines, tireless responsibilities, and the demands of our dealership — a mixture of both excitement and stress — yoga was always there to fall back on as an escape from a fast-paced life.

The day began like unlike any other — September 11th, 2001. But that day at Cadwell Park was eclipsed by tragic events across the Atlantic and will forever be etched in my memory.

Accompanied by my brother and a friend — both on crutches, recovering from surgeries — the air was charged with excitement. Little did we know that the day would demand more than just the thrill of the track. Firstly, only having just arrived, I found myself called to the medical centre. There was an emergency to deal with, as a friend riding one of our bikes had been knocked off. While we waited for the helicopter, my job was to keep him calm.

His refusal to be flown to the hospital was my first challenge of the day, but with broken ribs and a head injury it was vitally important that he be seen immediately.

As the helicopter whisked him away, news of the terrorist attacks reached us. We were hit by shock, horror, and a reminder that life's tapestry weaves together moments of pleasure and sorrow, often in the most unexpected places. The story of 9/11 at Cadwell Park became a chapter of unexpected challenges, compassion in the face of adversity, and a reminder that even whilst enjoying the thrill of the track, life can unveil moments that demand our shared humanity.

RACING HIGHS AND LOWS – FROM EXCITEMENT TO SORROW

The sponsorship of a super sport race team at the BSB (British Super Bikes) races was an exciting time. With our matching team race shirts, we became a tightly knit community, and I enjoy looking through the photos that provide memories of those days long ago. The journey expanded beyond the track of British Superbikes to the road at the prestigious Isle of Man TT, where we sponsored a team.

In the world of racing, participants are acutely aware of the risks that come with the pursuit of speed; the exhilaration on the track or road, accompanied by an acknowledgement of the inherent dangers. Racers embrace this reality with courage, skill, and an unwavering passion for the sport. However, the effects of these risks extend far beyond the racetrack and roads, touching the lives of everyone involved.

In amongst the highs, racing revealed its not-so-wonderful side — the memory of that day a haze of limited recollection, marked by the reality of our rider left in a coma. The narrative shifted from the excitement of participation to sorrow and introspection. The support that once surged with unbridled enthusiasm began to wane as the realisation of the not-so-wonderful side of racing unfolded, leaving an indelible mark on our team and my personal journey.

The chapter concludes with a poignant acknowledgement of the less glamorous side of racing, a moment when excitement turns to sorrow and the resounding effects that linger in our memories as a reminder of how quickly life can change in a breath. In its wake is a need for peace, a silent call amongst the echoes of engines and the uncertainties of life. Enter yoga — not as a physical practice alone, but as a refuge for the mind and soul.

The journey toward peace for me is ongoing, a continual evolution shaped by my experiences, a commitment to nurturing the soul and finding balance amongst life's relentless moments. Concluding with the understanding that seeking peace is not an escape from life's complexities but a courageous embrace of its many contradictions.

THE KNEE

As I reflect on the early part of 2022, my knee had finally reached its breaking point. The walks were becoming shorter and more painful. It was time to make a decision, and an appointment with the surgeon resulted in the wait for a full knee replacement. He anticipated a six- to nine-month wait, which became more like well over a year.

Faced with this extended timeline, and after a call to the secretary and a wait of now fourteen months, we decided to seize the opportunity for a month-long adventure. So, in June 2023, with our trusty campervan and doggy companions, we embarked on a journey across Europe, exploring the picturesque landscapes of France, the vibrant culture of Spain, and the coastal beauty of Portugal — over 3000 miles of winding roads, and the beginning of the manuscript which would eventually become this book.

I always miss my yoga teaching when away, so I left my classes with a short practice for the month. Little did I know it would find itself in these pages, but it feels like a great place to either start yoga or continue a home practice (at the end of the book).

So, I was then ready to face surgery with a mix of hope, weariness, and the knowledge that once again I'd be in the hands of someone I trust, and of course to the power of a deep grounding yoga breath. Sometimes, it's the small things that get us through the biggest challenges.

I always have bread left over when camping, and make Bruschetta as a tasty snack, or sometimes our main meal of the day.

My Bruschetta: Left over french stick, ciabatta, or rolls. Tomatoes. Olive oil spray. Balsamic vinegar. Onion. Garlic. Mushrooms (optional). Cheese (optional).

Toast the bread under the grill, or spray with olive oil and place in the frying pan. Pan fry the onions and tomatoes, (sometimes I add mushrooms), add some balsamic vinegar and garlic, place tomatoes, onions onto the bread, sprinkle some cheese on top, optional. Place under the grill. Enjoy...

SURGERY

Lying in bed, I'm held captive by the relentless waves of pain, each surge a throbbing reminder of the recent surgery. It is a symphony of sensations, aching, sharp, a dance of hot and cold. Sleep not possible, discomfort my companion in this restless state, I turn to a breath practice. Inhale healing prana, exhale discomfort is my mantra; this pain will pass, inhale positive prana, exhale pain. Each breath is an affirmation, a declaration of resilience in the face of discomfort. Inhale energy, exhale impatience, the mantra weaves through my thoughts as a thread. Endurance is a journey, and patience is the currency of healing.

The room is silent, but within me a dialogue between breath, mantra, and the persistent pulse of pain is interrupted by the sobbing lady in the room next door. Sleep broken again with another wave of pain, patience tested, a call to the nurse for pain relief, and a long wait for that elusive pain relief and all-important sleep. And so, in the darkness of another night, I continue this internal symphony of resilience and the belief that this moment too will pass.

As I continue to navigate through this period of rehabilitation, my bedside companions are more than just books; they are sources of inspiration and peace. The Bhagavad Gita, Patanjali's Yoga Sutras stand as a guiding light, offering encouragement when most needed. The Upanishads, with their profound insights into philosophy, provide a much-needed distraction. In the quiet moments of rehabilitation, I return to the Hatha Yoga Pradipika, unravelling again the teachings on asanas, a reminder of different breath practices, pranayama, kriyas, mudras, bandhas, chakras, and mantras. It's a comprehensive manual for any yoga enthusiast or teacher, illuminating the holistic nature of yoga. The ethical guidelines of Yamas and Niyamas — the first two limbs of yoga — encourage me to avoid violence, dishonesty, theft, and possessiveness, and guide me towards contentment and the pursuit of knowledge. These texts aren't just intellectual pursuits and words on a page. They are threads of wisdom weaving their way through my rehabilitation and offering a holistic approach to my recovery.

As I continue on this journey, I draw strength and inspiration from these sacred teachings, allowing them to illuminate the path to healing.

PHYSIOTHERAPY

My first group session after surgery was unfortunately delayed, because the pain relief side effects made me so sick that I couldn't leave the house.

So, a week behind, I face the challenge of the 30-mile journey to physio, upon arrival the walk with crutches then meeting others in the waiting room. They were all ahead of me in terms of recovery, all with different tales of their surgeries and individual experiences. One lady close to tears, while others talk positively about their progress.

The Physiotherapist takes me to one side, after giving the group the instructions for that day's session. She dives straight in with a measurement of the bend in the knee — not so good — explaining it will require a lot of hard work. I respond of course, I'm eager to regain my mobility, so I'm up for that. However, it's so swollen it just won't bend much. She measures how straight the knee is — top marks for that. *Great*, my slightly irritated inner self shouts. The physiotherapist, more than capable but lacking in empathy and humour, puts me to work then moves onto her next customer, who she manages to reduce to tears. No more 60-mile round trip to group physiotherapy for me, thanks.

I was lucky to be given my own personal physiotherapist, who gave me an individual plan, which was much better. However, no matter how hard I tried, how much I iced, and how much pain I inflicted upon myself, the swollen new knee just wouldn't bend enough. Maybe the bend I had achieved would have satisfied some, but I needed more, and after a check-up with my surgeon and a diagnosis of arthrofibrosis, further surgery was required. I was feeling very much like a failure, but I was encouraged by my surgeon that this can happen and not to blame myself, or listen to any negative comments, he would fix it.

What followed was another beginning, but this time with better pain relief, fewer side effects, and the torture machine CPM (Continuous Progressive Movement). I mention this not to moan about our services but as an option after surgery for those of us who develop a lot of scar tissue. The torture — whoops, I mean CPM — machine is a valuable tool for recovery. Yes, it's expensive to hire and arduous to use, but it definitely helped me achieve my goal with regards to the bend in my knee, albeit frustrating at times.

We are so very lucky to have these options and facilities available to us — the amazing surgeons, doctors, nurses, administrators, anaesthetists, cleaners, chefs, porters, and physiotherapists. Most of them do their jobs with a smile, and some with a great sense of humour.

MY JOURNEY FINDING BALANCE AND WELL-BEING THROUGH YOGA

Three weeks' post-knee replacement surgery felt like the perfect time to dip my toes into some yoga rehabilitation.

I started things off gently, just sitting in the yoga hammock, bending the knee, progressing to a forward fold with my foot in the hammock. Quite the milestone. Encouraged by my mobility, I decided to go for it and tried a supported backbend, which was surprisingly do-able, followed by down dog. I wasn't ready for any advanced poses, not ready to kneel either, so patience. I'd get there or not; my practice might be different but that's okay.

I had the underfloor heating cranked up for the next day's planned Restorative/Yin practice, as it's important to be warm. Taking it easy, I was listening to my body, slow, steady, taking one day at a time. For the first class back teaching, I went early into the studio and listened to some lovely mantras, then I moved to the floor and started to practise some seated poses, gentle forward folds, twists, and lateral stretches.

The return to the gym was a new role which required more words, less movement, teaching verbally, with deliberate pauses to guide, correct, and inspire. I found a unique fulfilment seeing my students move through the sequences, their bodies mirroring the postures I once embodied. My chair took centre stage, my voice directing movement as I spoke the cues, directing the ebb and flow of energy in the room, and a quiet pride swelled within. As the class concluded, I felt a profound sense of gratitude for the opportunity to guide, share, and witness the growth of a community that we had built and cherished over the years.

In the silence between words and the unity of the breath, I found a new dimension of achievement which transcended personal practice, a fulfilment in the collective spirit of a yoga community that had become an extraordinary journey of resilience and growth.

"Success is not final, failure is not fatal, it's the courage to continue that counts."

— Winston Churchill

LESSON PLAN FOR RETURN AFTER SURGERY NOVEMBER 2023

Affirmation: Doors are everywhere. I open them, and I explore with a fresh new perspective.

Start constructive rest, lying on the back, feet wide on the floor, knees resting together. Breathe deeply, eyes closed, hands on abs.

Window-wiper legs, inhaling and exhaling, allowing knees to fall from side to side.

Hug one knee into the body, inhaling, holding shin; exhale, flex and point toes; inhale, circling the ankle; exhale, hold onto the foot, and pull the knee into the armpit. Half happy baby.

Inhale and take one ankle onto the opposite thigh; pick up and thread hands through exhale, holding the thigh. Return foot to the floor; inhale, extend leg to the ceiling; and exhale, flex then point the toes. Lower to the floor and repeat the sequence on the other side. Exhale and hug both knees (apanasana).

Rock up and down yogic rolls, then inhale, rocking to seated, cross legs; exhale to laterally stretch, taking one arm to the ceiling then bring arm down to twist; inhale, forward fold, swap cross of legs, and repeat on the other side.

Hold onto the knees and inhale, straighten the spine, lifting chin to the ceiling. Exhale, chin to chest and slump, neck lock (jalandhara bandha), hold, repeat 5 repetitions.

Come to hands and knees. Inhale cow; lifting up the tail bone, and face, and dropping the belly towards the floor, exhale cat; dropping the tail bone and chin, pushing the spine towards the ceiling, inhale tiger — extending one leg and exhale, bend the knee and grab the foot with the opposite hand if possible. Repeat the sequence with the opposite leg.

Extended child's pose. From hands and knees, inhale, move the buttocks towards the heels; exhale, extend arms forward on the floor; inhale, onto fingertips and move to right; exhale, lowering for a lateral stretch. Repeat to the left. Curl toes and inhale; lift knees to exhale straight legs, downward facing dog; inhale, walk feet to forward fold, half forward fold; exhale to forward fold; inhale to standing mountain.

Sun sal B with warrior 1 2 3; repeat on the other leg. Flow with the breath.

Step to wide leg squat, elbows shoulder high, palms forward. Inhale, straighten legs and arms; exhale to bent knees and elbows. Straighten legs and exhale to triangle, extending arm to ceiling; revolve the triangle by taking the extended arm to the floor or a brick/block, and twist the body in the opposite direction. Repeat on the other leg. Add advanced pose half-moon balance to the sequence, Ardha Chandrasana. Bending one knee, bring the same hand to the floor and inhale, extending the opposite leg to hip height, then straighten the standing leg and inhale the arm to the ceiling, exhale down. You can revolve the balance to increase the difficulty of the pose. Repeat on the other side.

Flow to the floor, inhale sphinx, resting on the forearms, elbows under shoulders, palms down on the floor. Take a few breaths, inhale to sphinx plank, lifting the knees off the floor, with toes curled under; exhale lower back to sphinx, take a few breaths; inhale to sphinx plank, 3 repetitions. Move to hanging cobra, bend one knee and flex toes to the floor, push into the forearms and lift elbows off the floor, repeat with the other leg, then try bending both knees. (Don't lift elbows if you have a sore back). Then move into child's pose.

Seated staff pose, inhale to lift arms; exhale to seated forward fold, grabbing feet if possible. Take a brick in-between hands and inhale lift to the ceiling and exhale to bend elbows taking the brick to the back of the neck, inhale lift the brick to the ceiling and exhale to forward fold, taking the brick to the soles of the feet if possible, inhale back extending arms to ceiling and repeat.Supported fish. Take a bolster or blocks under the back, with legs extended. Open the chest by relaxing the arms down beside you with the palms facing up for 10 breaths; supported bridge, move the bolster or blocks under the buttocks and bend the knees with the feet on the floor for 10 breaths.

Easy twist on each side. Bringing the knees together, take them both over to one side, bringing the hands together in a closed twist, hips stacked; inhale, dragging the arm/hand along the floor above the head; exhaling to an open twist with shoulders on the floor; inhale the arm/hand back along the floor to the closed twist. Repeat 3 times, holding the open twist, extending the opposite arm along the floor, with the shoulders remaining flat on the floor.

Savasana.

Relaxation. Focus on the breath with eyes closed. Now visualise the number 30, and start counting the breath backwards from 30: inhale, exhale 29; inhale, exhale 28; and continue down to 1. Then allow the breath to simply ebb and flow, in and out, noticing how the breath now feels. The body now completely relaxed, rest for a few minutes, or longer if you have time.

CHALLENGE OF THE STAIRS

Looking up at the stairs, I can't walk up them unaided. The simple action of putting one foot onto the first step and then following through with the opposite foot... I just can't do it. I'm trying, but I can't. The knee just won't bend. I have no strength, no stamina. *Is this it?* I ask myself. *Is this my recovery?* No, surely not.

Nine months after full knee replacement surgery, four-and-a-half months after manipulation under general anaesthetic, I finally walked up the stairs one foot after the other without holding on. I mention this, because how can something seeming so insignificantly small mean so very much? But it just did. Another important milestone was kneeling. Yes, I can and do kneel on my new knee, but I use a gardening kneeling pad at the moment, which helps. There are some poses that I struggle with, but I'm getting stronger, and I know with perseverance I'll find a new edge; it might be different, but that's just fine.

Also, I'm riding again. I wasn't sure I'd be able to, as my present motorbike is a GSXR sports motorbike and riding it requires a big bend in the knee. But after a couple of short rides out with my partner, I felt strong enough to travel on my own to the gym — not without incident, but that's another story. These little victories may seem small, but collectively they're massive.

So, to anyone going through any kind of rehabilitation, don't compare yourself to anyone else. Your recovery is like you, individual and unique. Take your time, be kind to yourself, be patient, have faith, and you'll get there eventually.

"You never know how strong you are until being strong is your only choice."

—Bob Marley

FIRST LONG HAUL SINCE COVID AND SURGERY

JAMAICA 2024, and the perfect escape. Caribbean sun, clear blue warm sea, and beautiful sandy beaches — paradise, with the added laid-back vibe of the Jamaican people lending itself to long days of relaxation, interspersed with yoga and water sports.

Long haul flights are always a challenge for me, and unfortunately in economy the seats are really only big enough for one person. My journey was made that bit more uncomfortable by my neighbour's need for some extra space.

The long journey continued with a two-hour transfer along some truly terrible roads, full of massive pot holes and extremely heavy traffic, but we were rewarded with a wonderful tour of the island, eventually we arrived in our little piece of paradise — a fantastic room, a nice meal, and a huge, comfortable bed. The following day, with an aching body, off I went to the studio for my first yoga class of the holiday.

The teacher was from Europe, and although English wasn't her first language, yoga most certainly is. I managed to complete the class with only one modification. The following week, a change of teacher, Jivamukti, and a fortunate one-to-one was perfect and just what I needed. I was now ready to face any class with the confidence that my fitness was improving.

I had my first ever experience of parasailing, finding myself suspended 400ft in the sky, heart racing, yoga breath engaged, definitely out of my comfort zone, but well worth it. The views were amazing, and the experience most exhilarating.

The following days were filled with swimming, canoeing, snorkelling, and of course yoga. I met my much-anticipated return to snorkelling with a degree of nervousness and that strange feeling of both excitement and fear at the same time. As I was handed some fins, a mask, and lifejacket, in that moment I truly realised just how far I had come. Will's face was a picture of concern as I launched myself off the side of the boat and confidently swam around the reef, then I managed to climb back into the boat unaided — another milestone reached.

Finally, we faced the long journey home. A change to our flights meant we did not have the direct flight we'd booked but a stop adding another couple of hours to an already long journey, followed by a storm and the need to circle around the airport four times whilst being reminded of the brace position. Waiting for a slot to land, the wind causing havoc, I was holding on tightly to my mala, staying calm. No matter how prepared or experienced you are, travel still throws up a curve ball and requires a great deal of patience, as it's out of our control.

Nevertheless, I've already booked the next trip, and Vietnam and Cambodia await.

> "I am thankful to all those who said No to me. It's because of them I did it myself."
>
> —Einstein

STUDENTS

A massive shoutout to my incredible students. You guys are my rock. Where would I be without your support and understanding during these challenging times? Your presence in my life, both on and off the mat, have been a source of strength and positivity. Navigating this journey with your encouragement has made a world of difference.

From adapting yoga sessions to fit my current state, to your words of encouragement and understanding, you've been a crucial part of my support network. You all remind me that I'm not alone in this, and that there's a community of wonderful souls rooting for my wellbeing. Your commitment to the practice and the genuine care you've shown go beyond the studio walls. It's so much more than a yoga class.

So, thank you, my fabulous students, for being the bright spots in this challenging chapter. Your energy and support are simply amazing. I feel immensely fortunate to have each and every one of you in my yoga family. Here's to the strength that comes from unity and the healing power of a connected community.

A JOURNEY OF INSPIRATION

As my journals draw to a close, it marks not an ending but a new beginning — a journey of regained fitness, adaptation, and the exploration of a practice reshaped by a new knee. The chapters have woven tales of resilience, challenges, and the unwavering spirit that propels us all forward. If these words and practices have sparked a flicker of inspiration within you, a nudge toward the yoga mat, or a rekindling of an existing practice, then the purpose of this book is fulfilled.

The yoga mat isn't just a space for physical posture; it's a canvas for self-discovery, resilience, and gentle exploration. May your yoga journey, whether it be a beginning or a continuation, be a source of peace and happiness as you navigate the twists and turns of your own narrative. May the breath guide you through the challenges of life, the poses give you strength, flexibility, and stamina in equal measures, and meditation offer an inner serenity.

In conclusion, you are what you consume! In 1826, Anthem Brillant-Savarin, a French lawyer, said, "Tell me what you eat, and I will tell you what you are." The Bible says, "For as he thinks in his heart, so is he." Plato says moderation is the key to health. But it's not just about what you eat, I believe it's how you eat, when you eat, and what you consume, including media outlets, news programmes, films, social media, books, the company we keep, friends, and family. I'm not telling you what you should or should not do — that's your choice — just that I feel influenced by them all. What consumes my mind controls my thoughts, which becomes my reality.

To you, the reader, I extend much love and gratitude. Thank you for joining me in these shared moments, for embracing the highs and lows that I've shared, and for allowing the essence of yoga to weave its magic your life.

As I embark on this new chapter adapting my personal practice with a new knee and reminding myself of the continued journey that yoga is, I leave you with my blessing.

As the light in me shines to the light in you, may your yoga practice be a sanctuary, as it has been for me; a companion always there, and a source of enduring light illuminating the tunnel that is life.

Much love to you all.

Clareyogini x

HOME PRACTICE

Start on the back, easy bridge (setu bandhasana). Placing feet hip distance, draw them closer to the buttocks, and inhale pushing into the feet, lifting the hips off the floor; exhale, bringing the hips down, and repeat.

Supta bandha konasana (lying on the back in butterfly) — drawing the soles of the feet together, and exhale allowing the knees to open, inhaling and exhaling.

Inhale, bringing knees into body apanasana (wind releasing pose); exhale, holding onto the shins.

Inhale to happy baby; exhale, wide leg; inhale, feet together; exhale, hug knees; and repeat as many times as you want (lying on the back, bend knees into armpits whilst holding onto feet; happy baby — take legs wide whilst holding feet or legs; bring soles of feet together; hug knees into body).

Rock up and down. Yogic rolls.

From seated, inhale cross legs, and exhale twist — do each side.

Hands and knees: inhale, cat; exhale to cow; inhale to cat; exhale to cow; inhale to cat; exhale to cow. Inhale, extended child's pose. (Cat, push the spine towards the ceiling, tucking under the tailbone, dropping the chin into chest, reversing the action, lifting the tailbone and head, allowing the belly to relax towards the floor, then push the buttocks towards the heels and extend arms forward along the floor.)

Curl toes under, inhale and lift the knees; exhale to down dog (adho mukha svanasana); inhale, drop the knees towards the floor, pushing the chest forward with straight arms; up dog (urdhva mukha svanasana) and repeat sequence; down dog, up dog, down dog.

Roll up to standing balance: inhale, tree (vrksasana); exhale, take the foot to the side of the leg or thigh. Hold for three breaths then bring the knee forward and over opposite leg, with thighs touching. Catch the foot behind the calf, if possible, in eagle legs; inhale, arms across the chest and fold hands back to touch, if possible; eagle arms. Repeat whole sequence on the other side.

Mountain (tadasana) — exhale, forward fold, touching the floor or block with straight legs if possible; inhale, half forward fold, drawing chest forward with a straight back; exhale, full forward fold; inhale, step to plank; exhale, four-limbed staff pose (chaturanga dandasana); plank, bending elbows towards the ribs.

Inhale, upward facing dog; exhale, down dog; inhale, warrior 1 (virabhadrasana), stepping one foot forward, lifting arms to the ceiling either side of ears, palms facing each other; exhale, warrior 2 (virabhadrasana), extending arms shoulder high, one in front, one behind; inhale, arms forward; exhale, step back and lower to the floor; inhale, child's pose for 5 breaths, buttocks to heels and forehead towards the floor, arms resting beside the body.

Come onto back with hands on the floor beside body. Inhale and push feet/legs to the ceiling, balancing on the shoulders, place hands into the small of the back for support; exhale, feet to the floor behind head with the legs straight. Shoulder stand to plough — sarvangasana to halasana. (Miss this pose out if you haven't practised with a trained yoga teacher.)

Savasana — support under the knees with a bolster or cushion (if needed). As you lie in savasana, feel the weight of your body sinking into the floor. Notice your breath gently gliding you down an imaginary stream, floating, safe and supported, and feel the gentle breeze as it caresses your skin. Sigh softly. Inhale deeply then exhale through the mouth, repeating 3 times, deepening the breath each time. Let all tension fade away.

Now bring your awareness to your toes and work your way up the body, relaxing first the toes, feet, ankles. Pause, then relax the lower legs, the thighs, hips and belly; relax your lower back and move your awareness into the chest. Notice how the chest rises and falls with the breath. As you move awareness to the shoulders, allow them to relax into the floor, then relax the neck and face, and finally the scalp. Take a soft sigh, letting go completely.

Stay here for a few minutes longer.

Remember, if you have any medical conditions, please seek guidance before practising yoga.

And one last thought: remember the Buddhist quote earlier in the book. If you haven't got anything nice to say, say nothing.

DZOGCHEN TANTRA

As a bee seeks nectar from all kinds of flowers,

Seek teachings everywhere.

Like a deer that finds a quiet place to graze,

Seek seclusion to digest all that you have gathered.

Like a mad one beyond all limits,

Go where you please and live like a lion completely free of all fear.

ACKNOWLEDGEMENTS

A big thank you for the fabulous book cover images designed by Stewart Shield.

Additional thanks to Jim Counsell for further help with the cover layout and photos: www.designcounsell.com

READING LIST

The Bhagavad Gita, Jack Hawley or Easwaran

Yoga Sutras of Patanjali, Mukunda Stiles

Hatha Yoga Pradipika, Swami Muktibohananda

The Art of Hypnotherapy, Roy Hunter

Awakening the spine, Vanda Scaravelli

A Life Worth Breathing, Max Strom

Light on Yoga, B.K.S. Lyengar

Poetry for the Spirit, Alan Jacobs

Brightening Our Inner Skies Yin and Yoga, Norman Blair

Yin Yoga (Outline of a Quiet Practice), Paul Grilley

The Magic Ten and Beyond, Sharon Gannon

Insight Yoga, Sarah Powers

Restorative Yoga for Life, Gail Boorstein Grossman

LIST OF ASANAS

Full Forward Fold — Uttanasana — A standing pose which stretches the hamstrings and lengthens the spine.

Mountain — Tadasana — A standing pose which concentrates on postural alignment and a connection to the earth, focusing concentration.

Camel — Ustrasana — - A back bend which stretches the abdominals and thighs and opens the chest and neck.

Down Dog — Adho Mukha Svanasana — An inversion which strengthens and stretches the arms, shoulders, buttocks, thighs, calf muscles, and back.

Up Dog — Urdhava Mukha Svanasana — A back bend, strengthens wrists and arms, stretches the chest and abdominals.

Seated Forward Fold — Paschimottanasana — Stimulates digestion, stretches and lengthens the spine and hamstrings.

Constructive Rest — A restorative pose and variation on Savasana.

Knees to Chest — Apanasana — A stretch for the back, improves digestion and blood flow to the internal organs, also known as wind releasing pose.

Supine Spinal Twist — Supta Matsyendrasana — Stretches the muscles that surround the spine.

Bridge — Setu Bandhasana — Back bend that strengthens the legs and back, stretches across the front of the body.

Child's — Balasana — A restorative forward fold, gentle stretch for the back and ankles. Relaxing.

Cobra — Bhujangasana — Back bend, stimulates digestion, strengthens the back, shoulders, and arms.

Plank — Phalakasana — Strengthens wrists, arms, shoulders, and core.

Warrior 123 — Virabhadrasana 123 — Standing and balance, builds strength and tone in the legs.

Bow — Dhanurasana — Back bend, strengthens the spine, stretches the shoulder, chest, and quads, aids digestion.

Hero's — Virasana — Stretches the ankles, knees and thighs; single leg is an option.

Reverse Table Top — Ardha Purvottanasana — Strength building for shoulders, arms, wrists.

Fish — Matsyasana — Strengthens the neck, stretches across the chest and abdominals.

Supported Fish — Matsyasana — Restorative pose which opens up the chest and shoulders,

Seated Twist — Ardha Matsyendrasana — Aids digestion, stretches the spine.

Seal Pose — Bhujangasana with arms wide — Beginner's or restorative pose.

Pigeon — Kapotasana — Opens the hips and lower back.

Cow Face Pose — Gomukhasana — A seated pose which stretches ankles, hips, thighs, shoulders, and arms.

Monkey (Splits) — Hanumanasana — Advanced pose which stretches hamstrings and hip flexors.

Wheel — Urdhva Dhanurasana — A back bend, stretches and strengthens thighs, buttocks, spine, and chest.

Big Toe Grab — Padangusthasana — Strength and balancing legs and ankles.

Happy Baby — Ananda Balasana — Restorative, release in the lower back.

Extended Puppy — Uttana Shishosana — Back bend, chest opener. Excellent stretch for the shoulders and arms.

Straddle — Upavistha Konasana — Opens and stretches the hips, groin, and thighs.

Corpse — Savasana — Relaxation.

Cat Cow — Bidalasana, Bitilasana — Together as a warm up for the spine, improves flexibility.

Tiger — Vyaghrasana — Tones spinal nerves.

Triangle — Trikonasana — Strengthens and stretches the hamstrings, inner thighs, calves, shoulders, opens the chest, and focuses on balance using the core muscles.

Sphinx — Salamba Bhujangasana — Alternative to cobra. Easier on the back and wrists.

Eagle — Garudasana — Improves balance and focus, toning for arms and legs, strengthens ankles and legs.

Boat Pose — Navasana — A core-strengthening pose.

Four-Limbed Staff Pose — Chaturanga Dandasana — Strength pose for wrists, arms, shoulders, and abdominals.

Headstand — Salamba Sirsasana — Advanced pose, strengthens the neck, shoulders, and spine.

Shoulder stand — Sarvangasana — Stretches neck and shoulders, increases pressure on the thyroid.

Plough - Halasana — Stretches neck, shoulders, and back, stimulates blood flow.

Locust Pose — Shalabhasana — Strengthens the back and spine.

Dancers Pose – Natarajasana – Improves strength and flexibility in the lower back, legs, and arms.

Half Moon Pose – Ardha Chandrasana – Balance, strengthens the legs.

Lion Pose – Simhasana – Strengthens the neck and voice, helps to reduce stress and anger.

www.ingramcontent.com/pod-product-compliance
Ingram Content Group UK Ltd.
Pitfield, Milton Keynes, MK11 3LW, UK
UKHW040720020625
6184UKWH00045B/430

9 781836 152422